ME, MYSELF AND MY BRAIN STEM TUMOUR

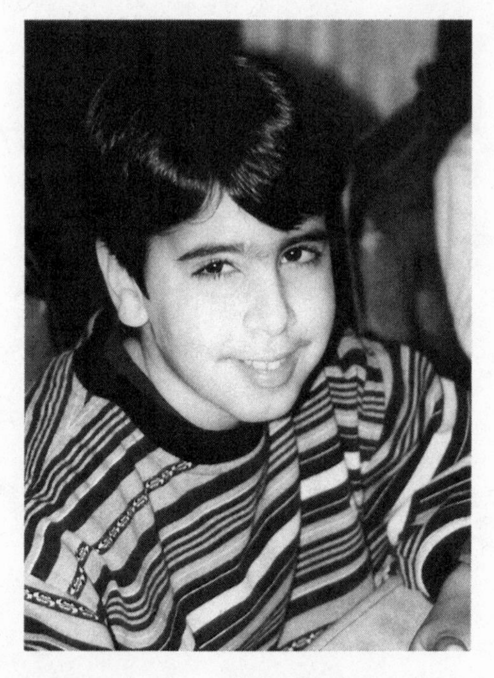

A picture of me in 1996 before diagnosis.

ME, MYSELF AND MY BRAIN STEM TUMOUR

Memoirs of a Pediatric Brain Cancer Survivor

BAYAN AZIZI

BAzizi

en EVERYWHERE NOW PRESS

16 17 18 19 20 7 6 5 4 3

Everywhere Now Press
www.everywherenowpress.com

Cataloguing data available from Library and Archives Canada
ISBN 978-0-9937147-6-4 (paperback)
ISBN 978-0-9937147-7-1 (ebook)

Edited by Michelle MacAleese
Cover and text design by Peter Cocking
Cover illustration by Kim Palmer

O GOD! Refresh and gladden my spirit! Purify my heart! Illumine my powers! I lay all my affairs in thy hand. Thou art my guide and my refuge. I will not be sorrowful and grieved any more. I will be a happy and joyful being. O God! I will worry no more. I will not let trouble harass me any longer. I will not dwell on the unpleasant things of life. Thou art kinder to me than myself. I dedicate myself to thee, O Lord!

(Words of Abdu'l-Bahá from the Diary of Mirza Ahmad Sohrab, May 9, 1914.)

Star of the West · VOLUME 7, PAGE 179

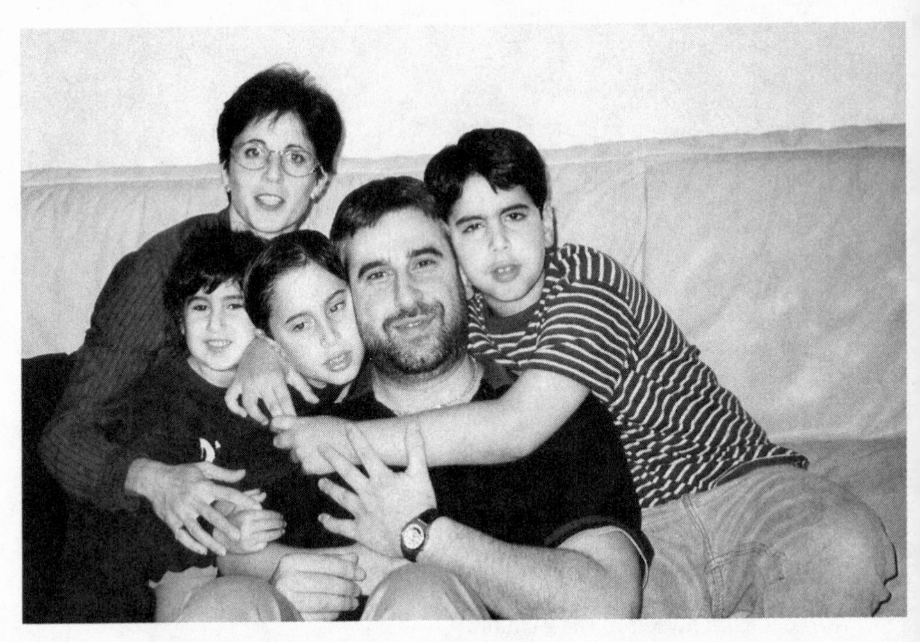

My family in the summer of 1999. *Left to right:* my mom, Nika; my sister, Maya (3 years old); my brother, Ashkan (7); my dad, Hessam; and me (9).

For Mom, Pa, Ashkan and Maya.

You have been there for me every step of the way.

CONTENTS

PART TWO: **A WISH COME TRUE**

PART THREE: **WHEN THE GOING GETS TOUGH, THE TOUGH GET GOING**

ACKNOWLEDGEMENTS

IT TAKES A real team of talent to write and complete a successful book and I would like to thank everyone who has joined me in working on this project. Lorraine Argotoff, Tricia Finn and Claudia Casper were all very encouraging and helped immensely during the initial stages of writing and editing this book. I would also like to thank Jesse Finkelstein and her entire team of editors and publishers at Page Two Strategies for all of their advice and support. My family and friends have made a tremendous number of contributions towards this book. Thank you all for everything.

PREFACE

IN 1999 AT age nine years, Bayan Azizi was diagnosed with cervicomedullary ganglioglioma. Cervicomedullary ganglioglioma is a challenging disease, representing less than 3 percent of childhood brain tumours. Although benign, this tumour exists in such a critical location of the brain that it is often difficult to cure and at the same time preserve essential brain function.

The cervicomedullary region is a small area of the brain that contains critical pathways controlling breathing, heart rate, swallowing, speech, movement and sensation of the arms and legs. A tumour in this area is impossible to remove completely even with the most sophisticated surgical techniques available today without causing serious injury.

Radiation therapy can be a useful additional modality of therapy to prevent the tumour from progressing and to induce shrinkage and senescence, however it is not always successful. Radiation has inherent risks, injuring both tumour tissue and normal tissue within its pathway, not only in the primary area of interest where the tumour is enmeshed with normal brain tissue, but also to a lesser degree it impacts the growth of important surrounding structures in the brain, bones, and soft tissue thereby affecting the person for life.

Chemotherapy has a modest role in the treatment of benign gliomas, in that it can induce shrinkage in up to 50 percent of patients and senescence in up to 70 percent for a period of time. In children this can be particularly valuable to delay the administration of radiation to the developing brain, and thus diminish long-term side effects. New research is identifying that specific genetic mutations play a role in the growth of certain gangliogliomas, leading to ramping up of molecular pathways that trigger tumour growth. Thus specific targeted therapy to inhibit such pathways and stop tumour growth is currently being evaluated in clinical trials. Such treatment may provide a viable strategy to combat this tumour and in tandem maintain the best possible brain function in the future.

The development of more sophisticated surgical and radiation techniques is key to improving the cure rate. Certainly there have been major strides to allow safer surgery and radiation since Bayan's diagnosis. Ongoing research to understand brain tumours and clinical trials developing new therapeutic approaches are paramount to allowing us to improve the lives and the cure rate of children with brain tumours.

I still remember the first time I met Bayan as a child when he had some mild weakness and swallowing difficulties. It was immediately apparent that his family were very caring and thoughtful and would leave no stone unturned to ensure the best treatment for their son. They understood the challenges he faced and would be there for him every step of the way. Throughout his treatment Bayan has persevered with incredible dignity and courage in the face of progressive loss of abilities and increasing dependence. It is heartbreaking to see a child no longer able to run around and play, learn with his friends, participate in conversation easily, enjoy meals and breathe independently. In spite of these losses during his teenage years Bayan has worked hard to embrace life, maximize his abilities and contribute to his community. His resilience is unwavering and a testament to the love and solidarity of his family and community. Bayan is an inspiration to us all.

DR. JULIETTE HUKIN
Pediatric Neurologist and Neuro-Oncologist
MBBS; FRCPC in pediatrics and neurology
Director of the Pediatric Neuro-Oncology Program, B.C. Children's Hospital
Clinical Associate Professor at the University of British Columbia

FOREWORD

WHEN I WAS seven years old, my big brother was diagnosed with a brain tumour. At the time, I had no idea what a tumour was or the impact this small mass on my brother's brain stem would have on our family. From the very beginning, though, I did know that Bayan's life was at risk, and this thought always has, and always will terrify me. My parents did all that they could not to scare us and to keep us positive, but there was no way to completely shield us from the gravity of Bayan's situation. Sixteen years ago, when I was seven years old, and he was leaving for Toronto to have his first surgery, I told him that I was willing to give my life for him to come home. I was afraid that I would lose my big brother, the person I felt the closest to. I couldn't imagine life without him, and to this day, when I look back at everything that has happened, knowing how many times we were so close to losing Bayan, that is one of the most heartbreaking and upsetting things I ever think about.

Bayan and I were always very close as children, and even though we couldn't be more different, I looked up to him more than anyone in my life. We would play baseball with my dad in the backyard, road hockey together in front of our house, wrestle and cause trouble as most young boys do. When he went to Toronto for six weeks with my mom and dad, my little sister Maya and I stayed with my grandma and it was around this time that he and I started drifting apart. After Bayan got back from Toronto, it was clear our relationship had changed so much from before his diagnosis. We weren't nearly as close and I think we were both subconsciously apprehensive with each other. On my end, this was partially because I didn't fully understand what was happening; all I knew was that most of my family had been gone for a long time and my brother came back looking and acting different. I became confused, frustrated and sometimes angry with the situation, with him, with everything. I didn't know how to express my feelings. I felt lost and helpless, and my defense mechanism was withdrawing within myself.

Despite my misplaced confusion and anger, Bayan has always been the greatest influence in my life and I have always loved him more than I can describe. After he came home, I became very protective and I remember getting into fights at school when people would make fun of him behind his back. Seeing him suffer or miss out on opportunities that would be available to most people his age brought me an unspeakable amount of sadness. I will never forget going to summer camp a number of years after the first surgery and sitting by the lake crying harder than I've ever cried because Bayan couldn't be there.

What is truly incredible, however, is the strength of character, resilience and immense maturity that Bayan has shown throughout his life. I can say with absolute certainty that I have not met anyone who has suffered as he has and who has accepted and made the best of their circumstances as Bayan has. Although he couldn't always do the things that others his age could, he has achieved more than anyone expected him to. Despite being given three months to live at the age of nine, undergoing three major brain surgeries, facing rounds of chemotherapy and radiation and missing months of school at a time, he survived. He completed elementary and high school, has taken numerous university courses, has written this amazing book and still goes out and explores more than I do. For as long as I can remember, Bayan has been the greatest source of inspiration in my life and I know that his story has already touched the hearts of so many. It brings me immense joy and humbles me so much to call this incredible young man my brother. I hope that his story brings you hope.

ASHKAN AZIZI
Kingston, Ontario, 2015

IT ALL STARTED on December 8, 1989, when another baby was born at Lions Gate Hospital. His face was scrunched up into a frown; he had big black eyes, thick black hair growing from his scalp, and chubby cheeks like all the other babies in the maternity ward. He would soon be cleared to go home to his family without any doubt in anybody's mind. That baby would be me, Bayan Azizi.

I was born and raised in North Vancouver with my two siblings, Ashkan and Maya. My brother, Ashkan, is eighteen months younger than I, and my sister, Maya, is almost six years younger than I. As of May 2, 2015, Maya and I live at home with our parents, Hessam and Nika, and Ashkan resides in Kingston, Ontario, where he is attending Queen's University.

I have overcome many challenges in my life, including a brain tumour, a very rare type of cancer that can affect all of your body functions and can easily lead to death. I was diagnosed at B.C. Children's Hospital in December 1998, and my family immediately found out that there was a possibility that

I would only live for three more months if nothing was done to reduce the threats caused by the tumour. But what made it even scarier was that the location of the tumour was very sensitive and therefore very hard for anyone to operate on safely.

When I was young, nobody but my family saw any signs of abnormality, except that I was often very congested and occasionally had a hard time swallowing. The doctors we saw before I was diagnosed with the tumour didn't think anything was amiss because I was growing at a normal rate. But as I got older, small signs started to become more obvious, and my parents knew at heart that something was wrong.

One thing that I have learned after approximately twenty years of going in and out of hospitals and doctors' offices is that although doctors may have university degrees and be experts in their fields, they aren't always right. Even though I am not a parent myself, I would say that parents know their children better than anybody else. My parents, for example, kept insisting to all the doctors we saw that something was out of the ordinary with me, but the doctors kept saying that everything my parents noticed was part of normal childhood development. That was until the day they found the tumour with a CT scan. Once the doctors found out about the tumour, they immediately stopped insisting that nothing was wrong and started treating me like any of their other patients.

Every night for the next little while, my parents put me to bed and promised that they would always be with me no matter what. The message I'd like to convey is never give up. Don't give up hope and don't give up on yourself. Sometimes it doesn't matter what the doctors say; even they can be wrong.

I was only twenty-one years old when I started to write this book, and now when I look back at my life I realize that I have always been a high achiever. I always did my best at everything and didn't let anything stop me. Even if I had set out to achieve a goal that was out of my reach, I still tried my best to achieve it. That's just how I've always been. And I have always wanted to be happy. I never let anything get to me. Even when my doctor diagnosed me, I didn't let it bother me. I knew my family and doctors would do their best to keep everything under control. I tried not to let anything upset me and just accepted things the way they were. You can do this too. Just focus on the good things in life and don't dwell on the negative parts.

Above all, I would strongly encourage everybody who reads this book not to limit themselves. If you do, there will only be so much you can accomplish. Work hard and strive forward until you have achieved your goal. Another piece to the puzzle is to see problems as challenges. A problem is a struggle you dwell on and feel sorry about, whereas a challenge is something you can focus on and overcome.

PART ONE

THE FIRST SIGNS

1

FAMILY FIRST

JUNE 14, 1994.

The Vancouver Canucks had just lost game seven of the Stanley Cup Finals to the New York Rangers. Seconds after the final horn blew to signal the Canucks' loss, a riot broke out on the streets of downtown Vancouver as thousands expressed their anger with their hockey team. Overwhelmed with anger and disappointment, the Canucks fans who were watching the game downtown started overturning cars, setting their jerseys on fire and looting stores. What had originally set out to be a social gathering to celebrate winning the Stanley Cup for the first time had developed into one of the worst riots the city of Vancouver had ever seen.

The loss didn't mean much to me, considering I was only four years old and didn't know much about hockey yet, even though it was and still is Canada's favourite sport. I barely even knew what offside was! Those were the days when I couldn't stand to watch a whole period of hockey, let alone a whole game. I was more interested in my stuffed animals and action figures than anything else. I also loved watching all of the Disney movies we had and learning how to read all of my favourite books. I especially enjoyed reading Dr. Seuss's books, especially *Green Eggs and Ham* and *The Lorax*; I would read those ones quite frequently.

My mother, Nika, was not upset at all about the game, considering she had never been a hockey fan. She was too busy with household chores and raising her kids to be involved with sports. She seemed to be competing with herself by taking care of my younger brother, Ashkan, and me as best she could. My mom would always make sure we washed our hands during the day and ate our vegetables at dinnertime instead of the salty chips we would snack on with our dad. She would even hide zucchini in our banana bread to make sure we ate healthily.

My father, Hessam, however, was holding back his emotions as he watched the Canucks march their way back to their dressing room. Ever since my parents decided to settle in Vancouver in 1986, my dad has been a strong believer in the sport of ice hockey, and he has taught me a lot of what I know about it. I still remember the days when he was teaching me how one team had the advantage when they were on the power play.

Every evening, my dad would play computer games or watch television as his way of relaxing after a long day at work. He would occasionally bring home movies on Friday nights to watch on the weekends. They were usually comedies, for as far as movies went, comedies were the preferable choice so that the whole family could enjoy them. That was back when we were still renting VHS movies from the video store. These days, we just get our movies off of the TV itself.

While I was watching hockey on TV with my dad, Ashkan was sitting on the stairs of our house on Violet Street in North Vancouver, wondering how to tear apart the Lego structure we had put together. He was always very physical when he was growing up. If you gave Ashkan a Rubik's Cube, he would try to figure out how to break it instead of figuring out how to solve it. He was almost three years old by then but was always a hassle for my parents. They had to clean up after him when he was finished making a mess by throwing everything around and breaking all of his toys. My mother always encouraged peace and joyfulness and never bought any violent toys or games, but whenever she brought something new into the house, Ashkan would do his best to turn it into some kind of destructive tool.

Not to mention the many times Ashkan bit me. Sometimes, when he got mad at me, he used to treat me as though I were some kind of chew toy. He would bite me with utter rage countless times. Once, he even made my back bleed when we were fighting over who got first dibs on the TV remote. And that wasn't all. One time, when my mom's cousin came to visit from California, Ashkan was so aggressive he almost took my cousin's eye out with a knife—but at least it was only a fruit knife. To be fair, he did it to save me. You see, my mom's cousin was trying to embarrass me in front of my family by pulling my pants down and my little brother, who loved me so much, came to my rescue, so I shouldn't complain about him too much.

About a month after the hockey game, after everyone had cooled down about the loss, my mom decided to take Ashkan and me to the park. We were all dressed in shorts and T-shirts because of how hot it was outside. Mom was pushing me on the swing set when something happened; I fainted and fell backwards onto my head. It was obvious that I hadn't just slipped but had lost consciousness, too. A couple of people saw this, and they instantly rushed to my aid. A little while later, I woke up in my mom's arms, feeling kind of dizzy. The fall sure did hurt a lot, but we went home and everything seemed to get better.

This was not the first time this had happened, and it would not be the last.

A few weeks later, we all went to a recreational centre to go swimming and sit in the hot tub. It was very warm and humid in the rec centre, especially in the hot tub, just like it was at the park. When we got out of the water, a similar incident happened; I fainted again, but this time I wasn't waking up. So my dad called an ambulance, but by the time the paramedics arrived, I had regained consciousness and was walking again. The paramedics quickly looked me over and said I didn't need to go to the hospital.

The medical professionals simply thought I was too sensitive to the heat. But my parents were starting to get suspicious about these fainting episodes, and they were concerned about my health. I had a history of fainting, dating back to when I was only a year old, and though unexplained, you'd have to say this wasn't normal.

So they made an appointment to see our family doctor, Dr. Neil, a general practitioner. He assessed me and did a bunch of tests, getting me to follow his finger with my eyes and having me touch my nose and then his finger. After the surprisingly short appointment, Dr. Neil said everything was okay with me and he didn't think there was anything serious to worry about. In my mom's eyes, Dr. Neil's quick and simple assessment was not in the least satisfactory, but at least he referred me to a pediatrician named Dr. Johnson so that he could take a closer look at my health.

2

THE EARLY YEARS

FAST-FORWARD A COUPLE of years, and we moved to a different house in North Vancouver, not far from our old house. My mom had just given birth to my baby sister, Maya, and we needed a bigger house than the one on Violet Street, where we only occupied the upstairs suite and only had three bedrooms. The new house was two storeys and approximately three thousand square feet. It had five bedrooms, three bathrooms, a two-car garage and a driveway comparable to Mount Everest going uphill toward the garage. We actually had the steepest driveway in the whole neighbourhood. There was also a nice view of the mountains and a nearby beach from the kitchen and living room. It even had an extra room where Ashkan and I could play with our toys.

In this new house, Maya had her nursery in a room upstairs, whereas Ashkan and I shared a room beside her with a bunk bed. When we first moved in, Ashkan immediately called the top bunk. I didn't bother arguing with him, because I knew Ashkan would always get his way. As for my parents, they had their own room across from ours. And downstairs, we had two extra bedrooms for the exchange students we hosted. They came from all over the world and were usually in their mid- to late-twenties. Growing up, my mom had experienced living in different countries and with different cultures, and she wanted us to have a taste of what it was like to live with other nationalities.

The only thing I didn't like about this house was that it had its main living area upstairs. Most houses have their living areas downstairs, but this house was a little different. Maybe the engineers and architects who were designing and building the house were trying to take advantage of the view from upstairs.

Another good thing about this house was that it was within walking distance of Dorothy Lynas Elementary, a school that offered French immersion as well as English. My parents asked me whether I wanted to learn French while I was attending school, and I decided it would be nice to speak another language. I already knew how to speak English and Farsi, and I was slowly becoming more fluent at the latter thanks mainly to my dad, who grew up in Iran and spoke Farsi as his first language, but we all thought having three languages under your belt at the age of six would be pretty impressive, so I decided to start school in French immersion.

When I first started going to school, my mom drove me, but when I was seven years old, I started walking there with Ashkan, who also went into French immersion. We had two ways of getting there: "the up way" and "the down way," as we would say, for the road we took separated into two different sidewalks. One of them led to the top of the school, and the other led to the bottom half. It was basically just a fork in the road. The up way consisted of more traffic and strangers jogging or walking their dogs. The down way was quieter and, in my opinion, safer; there was hardly ever a car that passed by. So that was the way we went most days. We would pack our backpacks with our lunch bags and school supplies and then walk for about ten minutes every morning. When we reached the school, we would separate to go to our classrooms. At the end of the day, we would meet on the school's gravel field and walk back home. We occasionally ran into a friend who lived in the same neighbourhood and walked home with him.

My passion for hockey was getting stronger by the day. I had memorized the Canucks' roster with help from my dad and was buying some Canucks merchandise with Ashkan. I was beginning to collect hockey pucks with my brother, and we were stacking them on the bookshelf in our room. We also collected hockey cards and hoped to get them signed one day. Ashkan and I would set up hockey nets outside and play street hockey with our dad. We even went to a couple of Canucks games at General Motors Place with our dad. Hockey was by far my favourite sport, and it still is. Mom wasn't too interested in hockey, so she didn't come with us. Maya was just starting to crawl, and my mom was busy raising her. This was our chance to spend more time with our dad and for my mom to spend quality time with Maya.

Another thing Ashkan and I would do in our spare time was play baseball in our backyard with our dad. We had a lot of bushes in our yard, so we decided which bush was what base and went from there. We had a baseball and a baseball bat, so my dad would throw the ball and either Ashkan or I would try to hit it. We tried not to hit the ball too far, or it would end up in the neighbour's yard. It was fun but not as fun as the street hockey we played on the cul-de-sac at the bottom of our driveway.

As for extracurricular activities, I was taking karate classes with Ashkan, taking swimming lessons twice a week and playing the guitar. The karate classes took place every Monday at four o'clock at the same rec centre where I had fainted. We would train hard for one hour and do sit-ups as well as push-ups with the rest of the class.

I had just finished the test for my orange belt when Sensei Mike noticed that I wasn't kicking my right leg the same as my left. He suggested that my mom get me to work on kicking my leg and exercising it a bit more. We spent more time working on my leg and even made some private appointments with my karate instructor to help get my right leg as strong as my left. Soon enough, it got better, but why my right leg was weaker in the first place was still a mystery to everyone.

When I went swimming, I had private lessons with a lady named Jacquie twice a week. Jacquie took me into the pool she owned and first taught me to float in the water. "Everybody should learn to float in water," she told me. "It's very important. If you ever go out on the water with your friends or family and accidentally fall in the water you can save your life by floating and swimming to safety."

After I mastered floating in the water, I learned the front crawl. While I was trying this, Jacquie also noticed a weakness in my right leg and told me that I had to work on improving it. I felt that I was using both legs equally, but Jacquie noticed that something was different with my right one. I told her that I would do my best to strengthen it so that both of my legs would be as strong as each other. I constantly wanted to go back to the pool and swim all day, especially to work on strengthening my leg.

My parents gave me the idea of learning to play an instrument, and I decided that I wanted to learn to play the guitar. I liked the sound the strings made, and I wanted to be able to make that sound. A guitar was also portable, so I could take it almost anywhere I went, whereas with a piano I would have to stay in the same room all the time to play it. Some of my favourite musicians were guitarists, and that helped me decide which instrument would suit me best. So my parents enrolled me in a guitar class with around ten other students in it. We started by learning some chords and then moved on to learn short songs and some scales.

I would spend a lot of time in my room practising my guitar skills, but my coordination was so bad that it made it very hard to play like everybody else. It was difficult for me to hold down the strings and strum my guitar at the same time, but I didn't let that stop me from playing my favourite instrument. I continued to play just like everybody in my class even though it wasn't as easy for me to physically play my guitar.

I liked the music my dad used to play on the stereo in the room I shared with Ashkan. He would play a Chicago album for us all the time, and that started my interest in rock music. My favourite song by Chicago was "Look Away," so after a couple of years of playing the guitar, I asked Paul, the instructor, if we could learn it. But Paul told me that most of Chicago's songs, including "Look Away," were played with the electric keyboard as the lead instrument. They only used the guitar for the background music. This was a real bummer for me because I liked the song so much and I wanted to play it myself, but I guess you can't get everything that you want.

But we did get to learn "My Heart Will Go On" by Celine Dion and James Horner, the theme song from the movie *Titanic*. The movie had just come out in the theatres and we all went to see it at least once. The movie was such a big success that Paul wanted to teach us its theme song in his guitar class. I enjoyed playing the song so much that I played it at the school talent show and even took my guitar to my grandmother's house and played it for everybody there. In fact, that was the last song I ever learned to play before I had to stop playing the guitar for good.

3

STILL WONDERING

BY NOVEMBER 1998 we had seen Dr. Johnson a few times, but he could not think of any explanations for the fainting problem and my lack of coordination. After a few appointments, he and my parents noticed a change in my speech; they were convinced it was becoming slurred. Dr. Johnson referred me to a speech therapist named Joanne. She had short blond hair and looked to be in her late thirties or early forties. Joanne told me to always keep my tongue touching the roof of my mouth and to always keep my mouth closed. I did my best to follow her instructions, but Joanne was not seeing any improvements after a couple of months of therapy. She thought the problem was that my jaw was out of place, so she recommended an X-ray. We went to B.C. Children's Hospital for the X-ray, which showed that there was nothing wrong with my jaw. Joanne used a variety of different techniques to correct my speech, but whatever she tried was ineffectual. Joanne informed my parents that she had tried everything she could think of but could not find a solution.

In the meantime, my parents were noticing other symptoms, such as my sloppy handwriting and walking. Both were becoming increasingly less coordinated for someone my age. So they made another appointment to tell Dr. Johnson; however, his response was that these two tasks seemed worse just because I was a typical boy and boys are usually sloppier when they are young. These repetitive excuses my parents kept getting were starting to bother them.

Another thing my parents remembered was that when my grandfather was first teaching me to dress myself, he noticed that I would always fumble with my socks and that my coordination was off no matter what he said and how he taught me. After my next appointment with Dr. Johnson, when he reassessed me for the last time and could not think of any explanations for my problems, he referred me to Dr. Burke, a neurologist at B.C. Children's Hospital.

When my parents took me to my first appointment with Dr. Burke, they told him about my fainting episodes and everything else they were worried about. After a few appointments with him, he came to the same conclusion as Dr. Johnson. My fainting episodes must have just been a coincidence. The fact that my handwriting and walking weren't coordinated and my left leg was dominant over my right leg was nothing to worry about. He told us that it would just take some time for me to improve, and everything would be okay.

My mom wasn't pleased with Dr. Burke's dismissive attitude and asked Dr. Johnson to refer me to another doctor, because she was convinced there was more to the story. She wanted to express herself to somebody else who specialized in neurology and ask for their opinion. I was a little confused by my mother's request. I remember asking her why we had to make so many appointments with these doctors when they kept saying there wasn't anything to worry about. She kept saying something along the lines of "something's not right."

My mom's uncle was in the medical field, so she took me to see him at his house one day and explained the whole situation to him. After hearing everything that my mom was worried about, he suggested that I have an MRI done on my brain to make sure everything was functioning properly. We went to Dr. Burke to get an approval for the MRI, but he didn't think it was necessary. However, he was willing to do a CT scan. This was similar to an MRI, but a CT scan is better for examining bone injuries and detecting cancers, whereas an MRI is better for viewing soft tissues in the body. This was a big deal for me because I had never undergone any medical tests and just the words "CT scan" were daunting to someone my age.

So I was put on a waiting list for a CT scan. It took a long time to get that appointment, but as soon as they had an opening, we rushed to the hospital for the long-anticipated scan. Since this was my first time, the technician ran me through the procedure. I had to change into a hospital gown, and then lie in the CT scan machine as still as I could so that the pictures would come out clearly and properly. The technician warned me that if I made the slightest movement, they would have to redo the procedure.

When it was finished, Dr. Scott, the radiologist in charge of the scan, looked over the pictures and found something he didn't like. He found an extra piece of tissue in my medulla oblongata, the lower part of my brain stem. That piece of tissue obviously wasn't supposed to be there but it unfortunately was, and what it amounted to was very threatening. He didn't know exactly what it was, but it's never a good sign to find something abnormal growing in somebody's body, especially in the brain.

Dr. Scott did not want to alarm me, so he called my mother into his office. He told my mom: "I have some bad news for you. We've looked over the scans and found that there is something growing in Bayan's brain stem. It could be cancer or a tumour."

It was a brain tumour, potentially one of the most lethal types of tumours that could ever grow, especially in that location. There was a chance that the tumour could be benign (non-cancerous), but there was an even higher chance that it could be malignant and therefore very aggressive.

It's unfortunate that the tumour was so hard to find, despite the advice of several medical experts. My parents had known all along that something wasn't right, and they had expressed themselves to many doctors, but they all said my parents' concerns were unfounded. When Dr. Scott broke the news to my mom, it was as though someone had poured a glass of ice-cold water from the crown of her head down her back. It was devastating.

4

CATCHING THE CULPRIT

DR. SCOTT TOLD my mom that he would send Dr. Johnson the results of the scans so that he could go over them himself. When Dr. Johnson saw the extra group of cells in my brain he called my parents to come and speak with him in his office. When he told my dad about the tumour, my dad's jaw dropped. "I knew it," he said. "Nika and I knew there was something wrong with him."

That night, we all gathered around in the living room. We said some prayers and then my parents told Ashkan, Maya and me that they had something to tell us. They told me that I had an uncommon, complicated medical issue and that we would do some investigating to find the best possible way of dealing with it. It didn't sound too bad to me, but that's because I didn't know the slightest thing about cancer or tumours. I was only nine years old and didn't know much about any medical procedures. I was just a little kid, and I'm sure that it was the same thing with Ashkan and Maya. They were even younger than me, and I didn't think that they would know much about this either.

That's when my parents told us that they would be very honest with us about anything they learned about the journey we were about to go through, even if it was unsettling to us.

The doctors never explained their concerns to Ashkan or Maya, probably because my siblings were too young to truly understand the effects of a brain tumour. The only times my brother or sister saw the doctors were during their visits to the hospital, but even then they didn't really communicate with them. Everything they found out about the situation came from my parents, who made an effort to reassure their two younger kids that everything was under control and help them keep calm. This allowed them to focus on other parts of their lives and not to worry about me. They did, however, see a few counsellors or psychologists, who helped explain the situation. And they had some family therapy sessions without me to help settle everyone. It was very difficult to get everyone to open up and share their emotions during those family sessions because the topic was so devastating.

Another thing Ashkan did to help get over the heartbreaking news was go to weekly sessions with his elementary school counsellor, though the time they spent together seemed to cover unwinding and de-stressing, rather than deeply discussing his concerns. They would sometimes play cards and talk, and often the counsellor would steer the conversation towards topics that may have been bothering him. There were many occasions where I would join them and get Ashkan to open up about how he felt about what was going on with me.

Not even my father completely understood the extremities of a brain tumour. His first concern was whether I could continue playing soccer. The doctors had just found something that could potentially change or even end my life, and here was my dad wondering how long I could continue playing sports!

An emergency MRI was scheduled for the next day to take a closer look at the tumour. I had to lie in a machine very similar to the CT scan, and the technician had to lock my head in a helmet to make sure I didn't move. She said that they sometimes had to sedate patients for this procedure, but those were usually little kids who would squirm and couldn't sit still. The technician gave me earplugs to help block the loud banging noise the machine made and a buzzer I could squeeze in case I needed to call for help or get out of the machine for any reason. It took one hour for the MRI to finish, and when it did, I sat back down in the waiting room with my mom. This was just my first hint of how patient I would have to be throughout this process of having such a complex medical condition.

After the MRI, we had an appointment with the neurosurgeon at B.C. Children's Hospital to discuss how the brain works and how the tumour would affect it. Dr. Williams, arguably one of Canada's best neurosurgeons, told my parents the tumour was about six centimetres long and was located in the lower part of my brain stem. The bulk of it was in my brain stem but the ends stretched down to my central nervous system, which is considered to be the bridge between the brain stem and the spinal cord.

Judging by the type of the tumour, and the fact that it was in the central nervous system, Dr. Williams and his fellow physicians were able to give us a faint picture of the severity and complexity of my extremely rare case. He told us that he suspected the tumour to be a slow-growing ganglioglioma, a type of tumour that arises from ganglion cells in the central nervous system. The cells were made up of pilocytic astrocytoma cells. According to Dutch sources, this only occurs to two in one hundred thousand people, and the people that are most affected are children five to fourteen years old.

At least what the doctors found was a tumour and not cancer. That minimized the chances of the cells spreading to other parts of my body. But, what the heck, they were already in my brain, so... whatever, they couldn't have been in a worse location. Not only was the tumour in my brain, it was specifically in my brain stem, which is arguably the most significant part of the human brain. Since the brain stem plays a major role in relaying information from the brain to the rest of your body, any sort of harm to it could be fatal. Just imagine not having your brain stem; virtually your entire body wouldn't respond to anything and therefore wouldn't function at all. We had to be especially cautious of my body's automatic functions, such as my breathing, heart rate, swallowing and digestion, because the brain stem itself controls all of these abilities. Dr. Williams didn't want to operate on the tumour right away because it was in a very sensitive part of the brain and he didn't want to risk doing any damage to it. He also didn't think I needed to be operated on right away, for I didn't have any obvious symptoms associated with brain cancer. He thought the best approach was to sit back and see whether the tumour was stable or progressing before he tried to operate on it and risk threatening any of my body functions with the harms associated with surgery. My parents did not accept this approach and argued that the tumour had to be removed immediately. They had already lost trust in anything any doctors said about me, so they weren't convinced by what Dr. Williams said either.

My mother didn't want to share the bad news with everyone in the family yet, but she did tell her uncle, who had originally suggested that I go for a brain scan. He said he could put her in touch with some renowned neuro-radiologists who specialized in these cases so that they could take closer looks at the MRI scans and give us their opinions. When my mother contacted them and asked if we should sit back and wait like Dr. Williams suggested or insist on doing an operation, their exact response was "You're damned if you do and you're damned if you don't." That was when my parents really started to worry.

My family started researching different hospitals and surgeons specializing in neurosurgery and found out that the first surgery on the brain stem of a child was done in New York by a surgeon named Dr. Cooper. My parents were interested in him and were thinking of having him operate on me. They mailed him the scans so that he could have an idea of how difficult the surgery would be, and then we waited to hear his response.

Immediately after seeing the scans, Dr. Cooper replied to my parents, saying he would like to meet me. We got very excited about this and were ready to fly to New York as soon as possible. The problem was it was January 1999, and he didn't have an opening until April. He had just discovered a technique to operate on the brain stem that only he knew how to do, so everyone around the world was coming to him either for surgery or to train for this special technique. We didn't have our spot in line with Dr. Cooper, so we would have to wait a long time to see him. That was another reason why Dr. Williams was reluctant to operate on me; he didn't use the same technique as Dr. Cooper.

My parents didn't think we could wait four months for the surgery, so they did the next best thing. They sent the scans to the best neurosurgeons across Canada and the United States, asking their opinions and whether they would do the surgery. My mom and dad even mailed the scans to specialists in a few countries overseas, including Japan, Germany and England. All of the surgeons returned the scans and told us that they agreed with Dr. Williams, that I wasn't at the point where I needed surgery. The tumour was in too tough a spot to operate on without doing any further damage to my brain, and they didn't want to risk doing anything. My parents didn't know what to do. In their minds, they had a son who needed surgery as soon as possible, but none of the doctors they approached were willing to do it.

All save for one. A neurosurgeon named Dr. Rice, who worked at Sick Kids Hospital, in Toronto, said he was willing to meet me and see whether it was safe to try to remove or de-bulk the tumour with his team of surgeons. We all got very excited about this and wanted to celebrate. One bonus thing to having my operation in Toronto was that my father's aunt lived in Toronto, so we thought she and her husband could provide us with a temporary home while we stayed there. That night, we went to my grandmother's house to share the good news. We decided that my grandmother could take care of Ashkan and Maya at our house so that Ashkan could continue walking on his own to school. He had his friends close by and could meet with them when he wanted. Maya was still only three years old, so she would need to be taken care of more than Ashkan. My grandmother didn't have a problem taking her to Montessori school and then caring for her at home.

Before we left my grandmother's house that night, everybody wished me luck with the surgery and hoped that I would have a good time in Toronto. My uncle Ron told me there were plenty of tourist attractions that I could go see there. I hugged and kissed my uncles along with their families and my grandmother very tightly before we left her house that night. Everybody thought that this could very well be the last time they saw me, but I reassured everybody that I would be back to see them in a little while. Nobody knew for sure what the outcome of all this would be. Before I went to sleep, Ashkan came and hugged me and did not want to let go. He said, "Bayan, I am willing to give my life to make sure that you come back."

5

GOING OUR OWN WAY

THE NEXT MORNING, on a grey, cloudy day in the last week of March, my father drove my mom and me to Vancouver International Airport. When we got on the plane, I sat in the window seat because I wanted to see the city get smaller and smaller as we flew higher. I read one of my books to keep me entertained as I flew across the country for the first time.

My aunt Purie picked us up from the airport in Toronto. It took some time for us to disembark from the plane and get our luggage, but once we got all of that sorted out, we drove to her apartment with her husband. They lived in the middle of downtown Toronto, so the street outside was always busy with pedestrians and traffic jams. The apartment had big windows looking out onto the streets but only had two bedrooms, so I had to share a room with my parents.

Once we unpacked and got settled in, my mom got on the computer and found out where exactly Sick Kids Hospital was; she wanted to see the doctor as soon as she could. The hospital was not too far from Aunt Purie's apartment, just a ten- or fifteen-minute drive. Then my mom made an appointment to see Dr. Rice later on that week, and my parents made a list of their concerns to share with him. It included my fainting episodes, my coordination and all of the symptoms my parents had noticed since I was only a couple of years old.

On the day of the appointment, we made our way around Sick Kids Hospital to Dr. Rice's office in the neurology ward. There were two other doctors with him, Dr. Harris and Dr. Davidson, who were part of Dr. Rice's team of neurosurgeons. When my parents and I first met the surgeons, we all discussed the tumour and what they could see from the MRI scans. I also told the doctors about all of the dizzy spells I had experienced back in Vancouver and everything else that we were concerned about. After consulting with them for a while, the doctors asked that my parents and I sit in the waiting room while they discussed the situation together. They all agreed that the location of the tumour made it almost impossible to operate on safely; they had the same thoughts as Dr. Williams.

While we waited, my father and I looked over the *Sports Illustrated* magazine that was lying on the table in front of us. We wanted to find out the latest news about Donald Brashear, the enforcer for the Vancouver Canucks. Brashear was more of a physical player than a goal scorer and was leading the NHL in penalty minutes that year. We had been waiting for the doctors for well over an hour when a strange feeling came over me, especially on the right side of my body. I forgot about everything and focussed on the weird sensation I was having for the first time. I lost track of time and didn't know where I was or who was around me. Eventually, the feeling passed, and I came back to consciousness. I didn't know it, but I had just experienced my first seizure. This one was a mild, absent-minded seizure, but it was the first of many more to come, and they would all be different. At that moment, nobody knew what I had just experienced, so they weren't prepared to even call it a seizure.

After a while the doctors came out of their office, invited us in and told us they could try to relieve some of the pressure the tumour was causing on my brain by removing one or two of the vertebrae from my spinal cord and giving the tumour room to grow. They also told us they could get rid of some of the cysts that were in the pons of my brain. Pons are a band of nerve fibres in the brain stem that are involved in motor control and consciousness. The cysts in the pons of my brain would explain my difficulties with motor skills and the fainting episodes.

Apparently, this would only buy time and prolong my life, not solve the problem. Dr. Harris asked me if I had experienced frequent and severe headaches, which are a very common symptom with brain tumours, but I told him that I didn't remember ever having any kind of headaches. The same went for nausea. This was also a sure sign of a brain tumour. I had never felt nauseous before, but I did tell him that my dizziness seemed to be getting worse every day. So the doctors lent us a collapsible wheelchair in case I ever got too dizzy to walk. I didn't want to use a wheelchair unless I absolutely had to, so one of the nurses recommended that I keep my hand touching a wall to gain some support when I walked.

Dr. Rice told us that if they did the surgery, there would be pros and cons to it. The pros were that they would get a sample of the tumour and could potentially get a proper analysis of it, and the cons were that there was a chance that I would never wake up again. He wasn't sure whether they should even attempt to do the operation, so he left the final decision up to us. He also said that even if we decided to do the surgery, we would have to wait a long time for it because the nurses at the hospital were on strike and the ICU was full with other patients.

We took a taxi back to Aunt Purie's apartment and told her about the situation at the hospital. My aunt had heard about the nurses being on strike but hadn't heard anything about the ICU being full. She told us to take our time deciding what to do, for it was really a big and important decision. She said she would help in any way and told us that we were welcome to stay with her for as long as we needed.

That night, we all went to a Persian restaurant near Aunt Purie's apartment to celebrate the fact that the doctors were willing to try operating on me. We ordered a big platter of kabob with tomatoes and bread with parsley on the side. I really pigged out that night on chicken and beef, so there was no way I could have dessert. Uncle Sorhab, Aunt Purie's husband, wanted to treat us to dinner that night, but my mom insisted that they were already doing us a big favour by sharing their home with us, so she ended up covering the bill.

6

TOURISTS IN TORONTO

BEFORE WE HAD left for Toronto, we had made a list of all the attractions we wanted to see and everything we wanted to do while we were there. Niagara Falls was first on the list. I had heard great things about the waterfalls from my teachers and classmates at school. They all told me that it was a great sight and going there was a once-in-a-lifetime opportunity.

We all got into Aunt Purie's car and drove south for more than an hour. We drove down the highway for a while longer and I soon started to hear the sound of rushing water. When we reached our destination, we parked the car and started to look around. We took a tour with some other tourists that started at eleven o'clock. The tour guide said we were going to get a little wet, so she gave us some waterproof ponchos to wear when we went under the waterfalls. She explained how Niagara Falls is the strongest waterfall in North America and told us it is fifty-four metres high and more than ten thousand years old. When the tour was finished, we went to the gift shop that was close to the parking lot. I wanted some kind of memento from this great experience, so I bought a crystal ball from the gift shop. Then we started to drive back to the apartment to cook lunch. I wanted pizza for lunch, and wanted to order it from a pizza restaurant, but my mom and Aunt Purie decided to make stew.

I was at the point where the tumour was putting so much pressure on my brain that I was constantly dizzy; therefore, I was always knocking into walls and needed a good night's sleep. I was starting to use the wheelchair more and more, which was not my number one choice. I always wanted to walk, no matter how dizzy I got, but I knew I had to give up sooner or later.

Next on our list of things to do while we were in Canada's biggest city was to visit the Hockey Hall of Fame, but little did I know that we would be staying just around the corner from one of the Seven Wonders of the Modern World. That's right, Aunt Purie's apartment was only a ten- or fifteen-minute drive from the CN Tower, one of the most famous structures ever built. Standing at 553.33 metres, the CN Tower is one of the tallest buildings in the world. It was built in 1976 and remains the tallest free-standing structure in the western hemisphere. It attracts more than two million international tourists every year.

I wanted to go up the elevator to the top of the tower, but the doctors at Sick Kids Hospital had advised me not to because of my dizziness and the air pressure the elevator would cause. I knew this would be my only chance to go up this high in an elevator, so I chose to risk it. Sure enough, I got dizzy and had to come back down and sit in the wheelchair. In the end, we stood outside the tower and took pictures from different angles.

The next day was nice and sunny, so my mom wanted to spend the day outdoors, but I argued that summer was coming and there would be plenty of sunny days to come. I had a thirst for hockey come over me and I wanted to get to the Hall of Fame right away. My dad had told me that *Coach's Corner,* the popular segment on CBC with Ron MacLean and Don Cherry, was filmed in Toronto, and I was hoping they would be at the Hall of Fame at the same time we were. This would probably be my best chance to meet either or both of them.

Ever since I started to comprehend sports, when I was only a couple of years old, hockey was always at the top of my list, so I always wanted to visit the famous Hall of Fame that only the best NHL players were admitted to. I was so excited about visiting it that I was actually contemplating if the Hall of Fame should have been the first site we visited instead of Niagara Falls. My first dream in life was to be an NHL player and make millions of dollars a year.

The first thing I wanted to see when we got inside was the Stanley Cup, so we had to go down the elevator and find our way around the building to the vault where they keep the prized trophy. When we finally found our way around, we took pictures of everything we could, even though the lighting in the building wasn't the best.

Beside the Stanley Cup were the Stanley Cup rings that are awarded to the players and coaches after they win the playoffs. I didn't know that each player and coach got their own rings until then. The rings are customized to feature the winning team's logo with the words "Stanley Cup Champions" spelled out in diamonds around the rings. They mean as much to the players as winning the Cup itself. When we were finished with this exhibit, we moved on to see the other trophies that are awarded to the players individually. We saw a couple of other exhibits before we left the Hall of Fame but didn't see either Don Cherry or Ron MacLean. My dad had already warned me that they probably wouldn't be there anyway, but I was just being optimistic and hoping to see the two famous hockey legends.

7

SOMETHING NEW

NONE OF US had forgotten why we'd come to Toronto in the first place. My parents and I had already sat down together a few times and talked about the tumour and what we should do about it. We acknowledged what Dr. Rice had said about the possibility of me not surviving if the neurosurgeons operated on me. Did that mean if they were able to get rid of these deadly cells I would die? That didn't make any sense to me at first, but my parents explained that the surgery would be so complex and risky that if the doctors made the slightest mistake and damaged any of the vital nerves in my brain, those nerves would stop functioning and they would therefore be useless.

Everything had been sorted out for us at home before we had left for Toronto. My dad booked time off work and my whole family took turns driving Ashkan and Maya to and from school and then caring for them at home. After a couple more weeks of sightseeing, we got a call from Dr. Rice saying the nurses at Sick Kids Hospital had come to an agreement and were back at work. He also told us that he was able to reserve a room in the ICU for me to stay in after the surgery. We had already told him that we had decided to do the surgery and have the doctors try to de-bulk the tumour. This would really make it or break it. We were definitely putting my life on the line by trying this surgery. It was one of the hardest decisions my parents and I had ever made, but it had to be done. My parents had kept their promise to be open and honest with me and had kept me involved in the decision making. They noticed that all of my symptoms were getting worse since the doctors first found the tumour a couple of months earlier, and they would probably get worse from here if we still didn't do anything, so I absolutely had to have the surgery as soon as possible regardless of the risks involved.

Dr. Rice's secretary scheduled the surgery for early in the morning, so my family had a quick bite to eat after we got up and left the apartment earlier than usual. I was told not to eat anything, even the night before, because the meal would interfere with the anesthesia. Watching everybody eat at the dinner table while I couldn't touch the food or water was a little bit awkward for me, but I couldn't argue with the doctors. I was sure that they had their reasons for restricting me from eating that night.

When Aunt Purie drove my parents and me to the hospital the next day, we first talked with one of the nurses who would be helping with the surgery. She told me that the anesthesiologist would give me some general anesthetic to sedate me and put me to sleep for the surgery, and that I would wake up in a bed in the ICU. This was my first time having surgery so I was kind of anxious, but my parents convinced me that I was in good hands and told me not to worry. They reassured me that they would be waiting for me outside the operating room with Aunt Purie and Uncle Sorhab. My mom told me to close my eyes and say a prayer to myself, and ask for the best. My parents even said goodbye to me in case this was the last time I saw them.

When the doctors were ready for me, the nurse called my name and I got out of the waiting room chair and walked fearlessly into the OR. After I changed into a gown and was lying in the hospital bed waiting to be treated, the anesthesiologist came into the change room and poked a needle into one of my veins in order to give me the anesthetic.

While I was asleep, the surgeons cut open a spot in the back of my neck. Then they had to remove the C1 and C2 vertebrae from my spinal cord in order to get to the tumour. Dr. Rice had already warned me that if they had to do anything serious to my neck, the chances of me ending up paralyzed from the neck down were very high. Once they were finished with the vertebrae, they started to carefully peck away at the tumour. The surgeons only de-bulked a minimal amount of the tumour itself, but that's because they were more focussed on draining the cysts in the ventricles that were putting pressure on my brain.

Nine hours after I had the anesthetic, I woke up in the recovery room Dr. Rice had reserved for me. There was a very slim chance of me surviving the surgery, but somehow I pulled through. It turned out that this risk we took came out for the better. When Dr. Rice walked into my room, he asked me if I was feeling all right and if I remembered where I was. I told him I remembered that I just had a brain surgery at Sick Kids Hospital and I must be in a hospital bed. He was very surprised when he saw that I had full mobility in my arms and legs because he thought that by removing the vertebrae there was a good chance that I was going to be paralyzed from the neck down.

I told him I had a strange tingling feeling all over my body as if spiders were crawling all over me. He said this was just a temporary side-effect from the anesthesia and to give it some time. Then the feeling would soon pass, which it did. After I had recuperated, I was transferred to the ICU, where I stayed in an isolation room. I preferred staying in this room because I had four walls separating me from everyone else, instead of just a curtain, like anybody else who wasn't staying in an isolation room.

When my parents noticed that I had awakened, they started jumping with joy and tears of happiness started dropping out of their eyes. They didn't think I would make it past such an intense surgery. But I was sure the doctors knew what they were doing and told my parents before I got the anesthetic that I would wake up and we would all go back to Vancouver as a family. What really surprised the doctors and my parents was that as soon as I woke up from the anesthetic, I started asking if there was any news on Donald Brashear's situation. I was very alert for someone who just had brain surgery and was sedated for nine hours. Apparently, he was suspended for one of the fights he got into with Marty McSorley.

When I got out of the hospital bed, I was very unbalanced and weak, and therefore needed my parents and nurses in the hospital to do most things for me. They brought me my meals from the cafeteria downstairs and even showered me and held my hand when I walked. These changes were hopefully just temporary, and Dr. Rice said that by doing different kinds of therapy I would regain my independence.

Dr. Rice explained that by draining the cysts and removing the vertebrae, he was able to remove some of the pressure the tumour was putting on my brain. That was the doctors' main goal, to get rid of some of the cysts and give the tumour some breathing space.

As soon as I started standing and walking around in the hospital, I was forced to wear a brace for my neck to make sure none of the remaining vertebrae wiggled at all. Because I had two of the vertebrae removed, my neck was not as strong as it used to be and needed to be kept in a brace. It covered my whole upper body, and had a little slot for my chin to rest in. I was okay wearing it around the hospital, but was embarrassed to be seen with the brace on outside in public.

I had to stay in the ICU for another two weeks after the surgery for post-surgery tests and to make sure I was recuperating from the surgery normally. The doctors and nurses wanted to check for any side effects and look for any changes in my behaviour. The nurses took my blood pressure and checked all my other vital signs every day just to be safe. My parents were staying with Aunt Purie and Uncle Sorhab, but they came to visit me in the hospital every day. I also had a television in my room to keep me entertained for a while every day. I remember there were other young children staying in the ICU at the same time as I, but they were talking with their parents and recovering in their own way, so I didn't get a chance to really meet them or talk to them.

Dr. Rice advised us not to leave Toronto right away because he thought that the pressure in the airplane would be too hard on me. So we stayed in our apartment for a week longer with my dad's family. I would snuggle with my mom in her bed and for her it was such a relief that she was holding a warm body and not a cold one.

Finally, after another week in Toronto, we packed our suitcases and were ready to fly home. But before we left, I made Aunt Purie and Uncle Sorhab a big thank you card for letting us stay with them for so long.

8

FIRST IMPACTS

WHEN WE GOT back to Vancouver, we first met with our whole family and thanked everybody for taking care of Ashkan and Maya. We had a big dinner at my grandmother's house with all of my cousins and uncles and aunts. I told them about all of the sightseeing we did and showed them all of the pictures we took. I wanted them to be there with us to share the new experiences with me, but they were too busy with school and work to join us. My cousins and siblings wanted to see the scar at the back of my head from the surgery, so I leaned over and showed them like I had with my parents. I also told them about the basket of balloons my classmates made for me as a welcome-back gift that I had found in my room when I first got home. It had about twenty balloons all tied together, and all of my friends wrote a short message for me on the big card that was attached to the balloons.

Before I'd left for Toronto, I had told everybody at school about the tumour and that I had to go across the country to get it checked out. My classmates all wrote me individual cards wishing me luck with the surgery and the recuperation. Even my teachers made me a card, reassuring me not to worry about the amount of schoolwork I'd be missing. They said that I was doing well in school and would likely move on to the next grade with my peers. I have had a great group of friends growing up. They have all been very understanding and supportive of me during my entire journey.

It was around this time that Ashkan started to pull away from me. There were a couple of reasons for this. First, we had spent so much time apart, and second, maybe he felt like he was being left behind because I was always busy going to doctors' appointments with my parents. We were used to spending so much time together and doing everything with each other, but now things were changing.

My relationship with Ashkan has gone through many stages, and it has thoroughly changed because of everything we've been through. When we were younger, we were very close, even though we had completely opposite personalities. I was the bookworm of the family, and Ashkan was the crazy daredevil. But we always looked out for each other, especially during hard times. As we grew up, we became even closer.

I went back to school with a nurse assigned to me from one of the agencies that provided care for people with special needs. At first, I had three nurses working with me on separate days of the week. Their names were Judy, Karen and Donelda. Judy came to care for me on Mondays and Tuesdays, then I had Karen on Wednesdays, and I finished the week with Donelda on Thursdays and Fridays. I didn't have any nursing coverage on the weekends or on holidays, because I was with my parents and they could attend to me if I needed something.

Going to school with a nurse was similar to a nanny taking care of a young child. I had to get used to being with them all day and to trusting them with my life. There were a lot of losses that came out of being with a nurse at school, such as loss of independence, which was very important to me. I also lost some of my privacy, but that's where the trust came in. However, I did meet new people and make new friends. I also learned some more medical information, even though the doctors had taught me a lot while I was in the hospital. But bottom line, I really didn't like having the nurses with me all day. None of the other kids had any "adults" with them at school, so I felt like I really stood out.

When I was with Judy, I liked to take advantage of her by purposely dropping my school supplies from my desk and getting her to pick them up for me. I wanted to make it as hard as possible for her to take care of me. I acted as though she was my maid and I had the authority to do whatever I wanted to her. I used to yell at her and say, "What do you think you're here for?" She would just say, "I'm here to take care of you, not to clean up after you." Judy would get me back by doing her embarrassing yoga poses beside me at recess or during lunch time. She said that this was her way of exercising during the day. But we finally called a truce that if I stopped throwing my pencils and papers around, she would stop embarrassing me by standing beside me and doing her daily yoga stretches.

The funny thing about Karen was that her son was in my class, so it must have been awkward for him to have his mother be in his classroom with him. I once asked Karen if she could wait in the hallway outside the classroom, and not sit with me unless I needed her, but she said she had to be with me at all times in case any kind of emergency occurred. But at least she only worked with me one day a week and the school year was almost over when she started working with me, so I hoped my friend wasn't too embarrassed by his mom.

One of the challenges the nurses had when caring for me at school was that I was still able-bodied and could, therefore, run around the schoolyard with my classmates at recess or lunch-time, even though I wasn't as physically stable as them. The nurses kept telling me that they had to stay close to me, but I didn't feel like I needed any medical help. Luckily, the school had some staff members and parents who would monitor the kids while they were outside, so they too would keep an eye on me and report on my whereabouts to the nurses.

Another problem we had was my neck brace. I really didn't want to wear it at school, because I knew it made me stand out and perspire a lot, but my parents and the nurses said it was the doctor's orders and I had to keep wearing it whether I liked it or not. I never liked staying in the heat, and when I did, the brace just made me more uncomfortable because of how thick it was.

Even though we had done the surgery on my tumour, we still had some other medical issues to consider. My parents told Dr. Johnson about the vertebrae that had been removed from my neck and asked him to refer me to other specialists to take care of that. One was Corine van Doorn, a neurophysiotherapist who worked at Hollyburn Physiotherapy Clinic in West Vancouver, and the other was Dr. Robinson, an orthopedic surgeon at B.C. Children's Hospital. Dr. Johnson knew we couldn't get any better than Dr. Robinson, for he was the head of orthopedics in all of British Columbia.

When we went to have our first appointment with Dr. Robinson, he did a CT scan on my neck to confirm the severity of my situation. When he saw the results, he said he wanted to fuse my neck, in other words blend it together, because he thought it was too weak to be left without support. He explained that if he did this, I would have limited movement in my neck because he would have to insert some metal rods into the upper part of my spinal cord to keep my neck from moving. I wouldn't have any range of motion in it and it could get stiff very easily. He was sure that this would be hard on me, so he didn't want to jump to a decision and do the surgery right away. Another downside to doing surgery and fusing my neck was that the rods would eventually wear out, so he or another orthopedic surgeon would have to redo the procedure and reinsert the rods several times over the course of my life.

However, there would be one positive result of the surgery: Dr. Robinson would feel reassured of my safety. My neck would be stronger than everyone else's, and I wouldn't need any support for it, so I could get rid of my uncomfortable neck brace right away. I also wouldn't have any chance of getting whiplash if he operated on my neck, because it would hold itself with the rods that he was planning to insert. After consulting with Dr. Robinson, I told him that I'd rather have full movement in my neck and didn't want him to do anything special for it right away. I was willing to wear my brace a while longer until we thought of another possibility for my neck and spinal cord. We finally left Dr. Robinson's office, and I kept wearing the brace around my neck.

The same day, we drove over to West Vancouver to see Corine for the first time. She worked at a physiotherapy clinic that had a number of certified physiotherapists who each did general physiotherapy while some also worked in their own fields, such as sports injuries. The building was very big, with multiple rooms for the physiotherapists to work in with their clients. It also had a large gymnasium with a lot of exercise equipment.

Corine was by far the tallest woman I'd ever met. She had brown hair to her shoulders and a heavy Dutch accent that I liked to make fun of. Corine specialized in treating pediatric neurological conditions by using neurological developmental therapy, so she was the person I needed to see. She had experience with chronic pain management using different types of meditation and visualization therapy. She also did massage therapy and acupuncture. This could come in handy in case I ever injured myself.

When I met Corine for the first time, she did an initial assessment and noticed the weakness in my right side, so she made a list of exercises for me to do so that I could strengthen the right side of my body. She had me stand on one leg at a time while holding weights and could see that I wasn't as steady when I was standing on my right leg. She also had me squeeze some putty to strengthen the muscles in my hands. I tried standing on a balance board, but that didn't work too well at first. It got better with a little bit of practice, but the balance board still wasn't my number one choice out of the physiotherapy exercises we did. There were also some problems with my fine-motor skills. To help the dexterity in my fingers, Corine would get me to pick up small tiles with my fingers and put them back in a box one by one.

After my first physiotherapy session with Corine, I went home, had dinner and had a good night's sleep after I had finished my homework for school. I went back to see Corine ten times for forty-minute appointments week after week over the summer, and she then gave me a list of exercises to do at home so I could continue strengthening my muscles and improving whatever I needed to work on. Every night, I practiced everything Corine wanted me to work on, and soon improved with everything, including the balance board.

9

NUMBER NINE

I STARTED THE NEXT school year the same way I had finished the last one. The same nurses still came to school with me. I was in grade five and Ashkan was two grades behind me. Maya went to a preschool in Deep Cove, a small community not too far from our home. I sometimes had to go with my mom to pick Maya up or drop her off because I couldn't be left alone.

One day in September, I went to Deep Cove with my mom to pick Maya up from school and we met a stranger there. This guy wasn't just any other person you'd find walking down the street; he was Brad May of the Vancouver Canucks. While playing in Vancouver, May was known more for his enforcement and leadership in the dressing room than for his scoring skills.

This was the first time I had met a professional hockey player, and since hockey was my favourite sport, I was very excited. It just so happened that Mr. May was picking his son up from the school at the same time we were picking Maya up. He had heard about my situation from other parents and teachers and acknowledged the challenges I was facing; my story really touched him.

When my mom and I first met him, he offered his help in any way he could and even gave us his home phone number in case we couldn't reach him on his cell phone. The next time we saw him at the preschool, he told me that he had a surprise for me. He went back to his car and got something from inside. It was his own jersey he wore during home games. He gave it to me and said that he wanted me to have something to remember him by. It had a special note he wrote on the back that read, "Dear Bayan, may all of your wishes and dreams come true, your friend Brad May."

The coincidence was that I was nine years old at that time, he wore number nine on his jersey, and it was the ninth month of the year 1999. It looks like nine is my lucky number.

After he gave me his jersey, I thanked Mr. May and we started talking about how much I loved hockey and how the Canucks were doing that season. I told him about how the doctors didn't think I would live for three months after being diagnosed and how they thought I wouldn't wake up after the surgery I had in Toronto. We talked about how frustrated my mom was when the doctors told us that there was nothing wrong with me, and he agreed that they should have been more cautious. He said it sounded like it really was a miracle that I was still alive and that I was a real trooper.

When I went back to school the next day, I started telling everybody about whom I had met and the jersey I just got. At first my friends didn't believe me, but I kept insisting that I got to meet one of the Vancouver Canucks and that he gave me his jersey. I ended up taking the jersey to school as proof. I made sure not to get it dirty, for this was now my most prized possession. In school, I was known for being the biggest Canucks fan out of my classmates, so maybe the jersey meant more to me than it would have to any of them.

I kept my new jersey in the back of my closet for a while, but then my mom and dad agreed that it was too special to be kept back there, and my dad suggested that I get it framed. So I went with my mom to a framing store and asked the man who worked there to frame my jersey in a removable frame in case I ever wanted to wear it or take it out of the house again. We took it home and hung it on a wall in the room I shared with Ashkan. That jersey holds a lot of sentimental value because such a special person gave it to me.

10

BEING TESTED

WE WERE STILL meeting regularly with Dr. Williams and Dr. Robinson to see if there were any improvements with anything. I really didn't like going back to the hospital so often but really didn't have a choice. It was like every week my mom and I would have to drive back and forth from our house to Children's Hospital to see either one of the doctors. It was like that building was my home away from home.

Dr. Robinson was still leaning towards the decision of fusing my neck, but I was sure that there was a way around this. One day, during one of our appointments with him, he had an idea that changed the outcome of my life. He suggested that I strengthen my neck with the physiotherapy I was doing with Corine. He wanted me to try to strengthen it enough so that he wouldn't have to fuse it and so that I would have full control of my neck. He had tried this method with other patients, and it had rarely ever worked, so he wasn't too confident that it would work for me either. But at least I could try it and see the outcome. It would be better if I could strengthen my neck naturally instead of doing surgery and fixing it artificially.

Dr. Robinson referred me to the physiotherapist at the hospital and asked her to do various exercises with me that would help strengthen my spinal cord. We all thought this was a great idea, so the next time I went for physiotherapy with Corine, I asked her to switch to working on my neck instead of focussing on the balancing exercises we were currently doing.

I met with Corine at different times and different places. Sometimes she would come to our house and work with me, and sometimes I would meet her in the gym at Hollyburn. We even scheduled a few appointments at school for after my class was finished or during the lunch break. I worked as hard as I could with her even though it wasn't guaranteed that I would strengthen my neck like I had strengthened my body.

Dr. Robinson was seeing a lot of improvement as a result of the time I spent exercising my neck with the physiotherapists. I would have to go back often so that he could do what seemed to be constant X-rays to see whether the bones were getting any denser and MRIs to see whether the muscles were getting stronger. He would do some other tests to make sure my neck was strong enough for him not to fuse it and maybe even for me not to wear the brace. I went back to see him so often that his secretary was probably thinking, why was someone with a brain tumour seeing an orthopedic surgeon as his main doctor?

Finally, after one of the X-rays, Dr. Robinson told me that because of the physiotherapy I did with the physiotherapists, my neck had fused itself and he wouldn't need to operate on it. This was a big relief to both Dr. Robinson and me, even though he was prepared to do the surgery from the day he met me. He was very surprised by my bone density, because this technique of strengthening your bones with physiotherapy was seldom ever successful. The only reason why it worked for me was because of all the perseverance, dedication and hard work I put into it.

This is one of the lessons I learned from all of this. If you set your mind to something, and work hard at it, it will somehow certainly pay off. Life is so much easier now that I don't have to wear a brace around my neck, and it definitely would have been harder if I had to have my neck fused. I wouldn't have been able to move my neck from side to side or twist it in any way. If I wanted to look to my right or to my left, I would have to look out of the corner of my eyes, or I would have to turn with my whole upper body as though I were a robot. I also gained some self-confidence from this experience, because you could say that I proved a doctor wrong. All I had to do was set my goal and work hard to the best of my abilities to achieve it.

We told my dad that nothing special had to be done for my neck. It still wasn't as strong as the average person's neck, but that was only because I was missing the two top vertebrae from my spine. I couldn't go on any of the roller coasters at the amusement park that was open during the summer, because the coaster would be going too fast and my neck wouldn't be able to hold itself, even with a head support. But that didn't matter much to me because I had already gotten sick a few times on roller coasters, so I wasn't too keen on going anyway.

I thought this would be it for me constantly going back to the hospital for all these appointments, but with my case, you never knew. Not only did I have to go back for more X-rays, but I also kept going back for more MRIs to check on the tumour. Dr. Williams ordered them because he wanted to make sure everything was stable and under control. After one of the MRIs, the radiologist who was looking over the scans saw that my brain had filled with more than one hundred little cysts that were putting pressure on my brain. Dr. Scott called my mom to tell her about this, but she wasn't too surprised, for my parents had already noticed that some of the symptoms I was experiencing before the surgery were starting to come back.

My walking was definitely getting worse, and it was obvious that I was starting to drag my right leg. I tried to focus on picking it up when I walked, but when I wasn't paying attention, I wouldn't take proper steps with my leg. I had been using cursive writing in school for a long time now, but that was getting worse no matter how many times I rewrote things and tried to keep my handwriting neat.

We also noticed that my coordination and fine-motor skills weren't as good as some of my classmates'. When I was just writing an everyday assignment, it would feel like I was holding something as thin and light as a straw instead of a thick pen, and I would sometimes have trouble holding it in my hand.

The big thing was that I was starting to drool in my sleep. My parents would put little hand towels on the sides of my pillow to soak up saliva and a tray beside my pillow in case I needed to spit in it at night. Just when we thought that I had the upper hand, everything was starting to go downhill.

The cysts in my brain were starting to multiply, and they were putting just as much pressure on my brain as before I went for surgery. Operating on them wasn't an option, and neither was chemotherapy, so the only other thing we could do was try to get rid of them by using radiation therapy. That meant that the radiation oncologist would have to prescribe the right amount of radiation and burn the cysts with a linear accelerator without harming me. A linear accelerator is a device most commonly used for external radiation treatments. It is meant to deliver high-energy X-rays or gamma rays to the desired area and destroy the cancerous cells without affecting the surrounding normal tissues. If the technician who was applying the radiation missed the cysts by as little as a millimetre, the rays would hit me and burn my brain, and that could be very dangerous.

Doing this treatment was another hard decision we had to make, for a couple of reasons. First, there was a chance the radiation would kill some of the good cells in my brain, because the tumour had infiltrated my brain stem. Second, there was a chance that the radiation could cause more cancerous cells to start. And third, there were a few side effects to worry about. We only chose to have the radiation because it was the most promising thing the doctor recommended.

So, before doing the radiation, the radiation oncologist and the technicians had to design a mask to fit my head and keep it bolted to a platform that I lay on so that I wouldn't move at all. We had to drive to the cancer clinic every day for about three weeks for me to get my daily dose of burning hot radiation. Considering how close the cancer clinic was to Children's Hospital, this neighbourhood was feeling a lot like home.

During the appointments at the cancer clinic, I got the maximum amount of radiation someone my age could tolerate, and when it was over and done with, we all blew a big sigh of relief. Getting the radiation was a very dangerous decision, but it was the only option left that may have gotten rid of the cysts. Even though there was no guarantee the radiation would eliminate the cysts, it helped keep them under control so that there wasn't as much pressure being put on my brain and I didn't have all the headaches I had before.

There was still one major problem. The tumour was still there and it was continuing to cause problems because it was regrowing.

11

RETRACING OUR STEPS

MY PARENTS WERE starting to get anxious about a difference in my breathing and swallowing. I switched rooms with Maya, so I now had my own room and Maya slept in the bottom bunk. My mom would sometimes check on me while I slept and she noticed that I was starting to skip breaths overnight. I was also starting to choke on liquids. My parents had to remind me to drink, because if they left me alone, I wouldn't drink anything for fear of choking.

So we made an appointment with Dr. Brown, the oncologist at Children's Hospital, to report these new changes. Unfortunately, he couldn't think of a solution and came to the conclusion that there was nothing that could be done for me.

We would not take that for an answer, so we called Dr. Rice, who said that he would be happy to see me again if we went back to Toronto. Within days, we got onto another flight to Toronto, and arrived there late at night. When we got off the plane, we took a taxi to a hotel and stayed there overnight.

The next morning, we went to see Dr. Rice at Sick Kids Hospital, where he had already operated on me with Dr. Harris and Dr.

Davidson. We checked in and were waiting for him in a hospital room when I suddenly stopped breathing and went into respiratory arrest. A Code Blue was called, so everyone who worked in that ward dropped what they were doing and rushed to my aid. I had maybe fifty doctors and nurses come at me, ready to do CPR or whatever else they needed to do to get me breathing again.

Thankfully, Dr. Rice was one of them, and once he stabilized me, I came back to consciousness and started to breathe on my own again. This doctor seemed unstoppable to me; it was like he could do anything for me just when I needed it. Imagine if this had happened just one hour earlier. I would have still been at the hotel with my mom and no one there would have known what to do except maybe call an ambulance. By the time it would have gotten to the hotel and taken me to the hospital, it might've been too late.

I was put into an isolation room after that and wasn't allowed to leave even for a minute. I had to have somebody with me the whole time. Everything was brought to me because I wasn't even allowed to go out on that floor or downstairs to the cafeteria. I would spend hours just lying in bed doing nothing but talking to whoever was with me and telling them how much I missed home. How boring is that? I needed some fresh air and begged the nurses to take me outside, but they said it was the doctor's orders to keep me inside because this could happen again in a blink of an eye.

My mom knew that I had had enough of staying in the hospital, so she compromised and took me out of my room one day to get a change of scenery. I wanted to go outside to get a breath of fresh air more than anything. But once we got outside, what did we get? A big gust of cigarette smoke! A bunch of people were smoking their cigarettes near the hospital entrance, which was okay to do back then but is now restricted. I couldn't stand the smell, so we went back upstairs to the ward. I guess I just wasn't meant to leave my room.

Within the next few days, the doctors came to the conclusion that the respiratory arrest was caused because of seizures and lack of oxygen to my brain. I was taking shallow breaths during the day and was skipping breaths when I slept. They wanted to try a BiPAP machine on me. The BiPAP (bilevel positive airway pressure) is a breathing apparatus that helps people get more air into their lungs. Dr. Rice wanted to try this instead of a ventilator because the BiPAP would not affect me permanently and it was a simple solution for my breathing episodes. The BiPAP had a little mask that fit over my nose and mouth and blew air into my lungs to help me breathe. I tried the BiPAP for the next few days, but it wasn't what I needed, so the next thing the doctors thought of was putting a tracheostomy into my throat and getting a ventilator to breathe for me. A tracheostomy is a tube that would have to be inserted through an opening in my trachea, usually called a stoma, or in this case a tracheostomy stoma, and a ventilator could attach to it.

Dr. Rice explained that if they did this, I would lose my voice and eventually have to stop eating and drinking. At first, I didn't believe him, because I didn't think there would be any other way I could get the nutrition or liquids I needed, and I knew that I couldn't live without them. He told me that they would have to insert a gastric tube, or G-tube, into my stomach and I could get all the nutrition and liquids I needed through that.

Would I have to give up eating and drinking? No, I would be able to make it past this barrier too. I was thinking that I had already made it this far without having to lose anything: it was well past the three months the doctors had given me when I was first diagnosed, I had survived the surgery that nobody thought I would wake up from, and Dr. Robinson didn't have to fuse my neck. And all the specialists I saw before getting diagnosed kept saying I was just an average person, no matter what my parents told them. I was starting not to like doctors in general by then, because they always seemed to be wrong about me.

12

MORE COMPLICATIONS

EVENTUALLY, I WAS cleared to go home and was flown back to B.C. Children's Hospital via air ambulance. I had to travel with a nurse so that she could check my vital signs and do other tests while we flew back to Vancouver. She made me wear a stat monitor on my finger to check my oxygen level the whole flight. The small plane landed on the B.C. Children's Hospital runway about six hours after we had taken off, and when we got out, I was rushed in an ambulance to another isolation room in the SNU (special needs unit). Travelling across the country from one hospital to another was nothing to be proud of—it was actually pretty depressing.

We told the doctors what had happened in Toronto and that they were considering putting in a tracheostomy because the BiPAP didn't help me enough. The reason they didn't do it at Sick Kids was because I would've had to stay in that hospital for a ridiculously long time to recover and it was too far from home.

The physicians at Children's wanted to see for themselves how the BiPAP would work on me, so I was kept in the hospital for another week with just the BiPAP machine helping me breathe at night. My parents told the doctors and nurses that we had already tried it in Toronto, but they wanted to form their own opinions. They kept me in the hospital for a week and then sent me home with nothing but the BiPAP, because they didn't think anything else was needed. We were unsure about this but didn't have much choice but to abide by the doctors' theories.

I slept all right at home for a few nights, but then a really bad experience happened. I had a grand mal seizure and stopped breathing again. My parents tried doing CPR but didn't know what exactly to do. My mother tried to do mouth-to-mouth resuscitation, but my mouth was locked and foam was starting to pour out. My dad immediately called 911 while my mom was frantically shaking me and screaming my name, trying to wake me up.

While this was happening, Ashkan and Maya were sleeping in the room next to mine. Maya heard my mom's screaming, woke up and ran to my bedroom. She knew that things were not right with me and was, therefore, in a state of deep fear. To this day, she remembers it as the most frightening night of her life.

Within minutes, two fire trucks came and then an ambulance. At that point, my parents did not know what else they could do, so they stepped out of the way to let the experts take charge of the situation. In the meantime, my mom embraced my dad; at that point she was sure I had left this world.

The paramedics injected me with something and then took me back to the hospital. Everybody thought I was gone by the time we got there, but somehow I was still alive. Whatever went on that night was intense, but I don't remember it, because I had lost consciousness before everything happened. That was by far one of the scariest nights of our lives. After we got to the hospital, my parents were very firm with the doctors and refused to leave until they were 100 percent convinced that my safety was guaranteed.

The doctors in Toronto had done a sleep study to determine my breathing pattern while I was asleep with a BiPAP machine, and it confirmed that I was skipping breaths throughout the night and was taking very shallow breaths. That meant that I was not getting enough oxygen while I slept. The doctors in Vancouver were still not convinced that I needed to be ventilated, so they redid all the tests that had been done at Sick Kids, including a sleep study, an EEG and diverse blood work, and still decided that the BiPAP was the best option. At this point, my mom lost complete confidence in the British Columbia medical system and stayed at my bedside all day and night. There was a visitor's chair beside my bed in my isolation room that could unfold into a mattress, and that became my mom's new bed. She felt that if she left my bedside, she would be like a fish out of water.

When I was still on the BiPAP at Children's Hospital, I was hooked to monitors that displayed my vital signs, including my heart rate and blood pressure. I also had an oximeter attached to my finger that recorded my oxygen levels and displayed them on the monitor in the nurses' station.

One night, the alarms from the monitors kept going off and they showed that my oxygen levels were very low. My mom brought this to the attention of the nurse in charge of taking care of me, but she said that there was a problem with the machines and they were not reading properly. The nurse casually left for her break and told my mom that she would look into it when she got back. My mom still was not convinced that the problem was the machines, so she went to the small closet in my isolation room and took out my portable oximeter we'd brought from home to double-check the reading. It showed that the numbers were exactly the same.

Within minutes, I went into respiratory arrest again, but this time my heart also stopped. My mom screamed and that got everybody's attention. Luckily, the ICU physician was in the room next door, where he had just been called for another emergency. He intubated me right away and got my heart going again. This was another close call, but this time I did not regain consciousness.

That was the last night I used the BiPAP. That was when I was transferred from the SNU into the ICU. Immediately after that, I started to get ventilated through my mouth with some tubes and became dependent on the ventilator to breathe for me while I slept. The nurses also inserted a catheter that ended in my stomach into my nose so that I could get all my nutritional needs through this nasogastric (NG) tube.

Eventually, I seemed alert enough to start taking occasional breaths by myself during the day, so the respiratory therapist wanted to start weaning me off the ventilator when I was awake. They changed the settings for short periods of time, but I continued to stop breathing here and there. I had to have the ventilator on a support mode so that whenever I stopped breathing, it would kick in and breathe for me.

I gradually started to become more responsive to my environment, but I was still dependent on the ventilator for a while longer. They had a television in the ICU, so whenever the Vancouver Canucks played, I would watch the games with my parents in my isolation room. The monitors showed that every time the Canucks got close to scoring, and every time there were exciting moments in the game, I would stop breathing. The alarms would go off and they would remind me to keep taking deep breaths.

13
SPUNKY

BACK AT HOME, Ashkan and Maya had been talking about getting a dog, but my parents were undecided. Since I was in such a critical stage in the hospital, and my parents were visiting me every day with so much on their minds, they didn't want the burden of having a dog to worry about. Maya knew that my uncle in New York had two big dogs and two birds, so she compared us with him and his family. She wanted just one dog to their two, and it wouldn't have to be a big one. Nobody wanted a bird, because it would just stay in its cage all day, so we easily crossed that out. My mom's big concern about the dog was the shedding and the difficulty of having to clean up after it with our carpeted floors. And walking it would be a hassle for them too, especially with all of the rain and bad weather we got in Vancouver. They thought a dog would bring in all the leaves and dirt from the forest we lived next to.

Ashkan and I had already had a cat when we were younger and we loved playing with it, but it ran away when we moved to our new house. My parents tried to persuade Maya to get another cat instead of a dog, because it wouldn't need to be taken care of as much, but Maya really wanted a dog. My parents told her how cute and cuddly our cat, Fluffy, was and that another cat would be just as good, but Maya stood her ground.

But then my parents thought that having a dog would help take Ashkan and Maya's minds off my situation and actually do some good. So they gave in and wrote out a contract with Ashkan and Maya saying that they would pay for anything the dog needed, including taking it to the vet and its food, but Ashkan would have to take turns with Maya taking the dog for walks, feeding it and caring for it. They were hesitant to agree to this deal at first but eventually signed the contract and promised to live up to it.

My parents wouldn't allow any of those big dogs such as German shepherds or Saint Bernards, because they would take up too much space in the house and they would shed limitless amounts of hair. My siblings agreed to look for a small dog that wouldn't shed, so their options were limited. I wasn't too interested in getting a dog because I was staying in the hospital and didn't know when I would get out. I had other, more important things to worry about than a dog.

Maya and Ashkan came to visit me with my dad in the evenings and on weekends. My siblings had done some research on different breeds of dogs and had found a few that would work well with our family. But we were all particularly interested in the schnauzer, a breed that originated in Germany and came in three different sizes: miniature, standard and giant. Apparently, a miniature schnauzer would be happy with indoor life as long as it routinely got some exercise. They usually come in a salt-and-pepper colour, but it is possible to find them with a jet-black or white coat. They are very good with children and have a lot of energy. They are usually described as alert and spirited dogs but obedient to command as well as extremely playful and very smart. Some dog experts believe schnauzers to be second in line to German shepherds in terms of intelligence.

The only negative thing about them is that they are known for barking a lot and may often attack other small pets such as birds, snakes and rodents. We were told not to let a schnauzer wander off on its own and to always be prepared for it to bark whenever somebody rang the doorbell. It was natural for them to be a little over-aggressive. Many will also attack cats, but this can be curbed with training, or if the dog is raised with cats. Our cat had already run away, so we didn't have to worry about her being attacked.

We decided that these were the perfect dogs for us. My cousins had also persuaded their parents to get a dog, so we all got into the car and went to get them from a breeder. I really wanted to take advantage of this chance to get out of the hospital and spend some time with my family. We needed special approval from the attending doctor to do this. He hesitated at first but then allowed me to leave the hospital for the day. We had to drive for about an hour to a breeder in Cultus Lake, who had eight or ten dogs that were looking for new homes. Ashkan, Maya and I wanted a male puppy, and my cousins wanted a female.

My parents picked out a puppy that had been born six or eight weeks earlier and had jet-black fur. It was playing by itself with a bone in the woods and seemed to be very cheeky. They thought that this dog would be a good match for us because it looked like it wanted to play all the time. He was also the brother of the dog our cousins chose.

The breeder told us she had named our dog Spunky, but it would be fine to rename him because he was still young and hadn't adapted to his name yet. We decided to keep the name for a few reasons. First, we thought that he was used to it; second, it sounded like a good name for a dog; and third, it suited his energetic personality. Spunky was a purebred miniature schnauzer who, like all schnauzers, had that cute little moustache around his mouth.

On our way back to the hospital, the dogs were starting to pant in the back seat of the warm and muggy car, so we stopped at a coffee shop to get lunch and to drink some water. That was one of the only times I got to set foot out of the hospital, so I had to make it last as long as I could by taking my time with my lunch and convincing my dad to drive as slowly as he could on the highway. I wanted to stay outside in the sun all day with my family and procrastinate forever going back into my isolation room in the SNU. When we finally got back to the hospital, my family dropped me off and I started telling all of the SNU and ICU nurses who were taking care of me about the new addition to our family.

My parents went to buy Spunky a new bed and some toys from a nearby pet shop, and Ashkan kept his end of the deal by taking Spunky for walks every day. Maya was in charge of feeding him and changing his water twice a day. Potty training was also an issue. The breeder recommended we keep Spunky in a kennel to make sure that he would not have accidents on the carpets. Everyone loved having Spunky at home, but the big problem was how much he barked. Whenever somebody rang the doorbell, Spunky always went crazy, barking his head off, but after they came in and he sniffed them for a while he started to cool off.

Spunky also had an enormous appetite. He would eat anything edible, especially apples and peanut butter. He loved peanut butter because it would stick to the roof of his mouth and he could lick it whenever he wanted. My family would peel their apples and give Spunky the peels in his food bowl. Whenever anyone so much as picked up an apple, Spunky was right there at their feet, licking his lips and barking, just waiting to be fed. We would also throw the cores outside for him to eat, because according to the veterinarian, they were good for him and would clean his teeth. We used this as a technique to train him instead of dog cookies, which are extremely high in saturated and trans fats.

14

DR. HUNTER

WE CONTINUED TO see Dr. Williams regularly. He told us there was the possibility of using chemotherapy to kill the tumour, so he referred me to Dr. Hunter, the neuro-oncologist at the hospital. A neuro-oncologist is a doctor who specializes in brain cancer, and since a brain tumour is, essentially, the same thing as brain cancer, Dr. Hunter was our best bet.

Dr. Hunter had just started working at B.C. Children's Hospital and I was one of her first patients. She was actually the only pediatric neuro-oncologist in all of British Columbia at that time. Can you believe that? The only doctor who specialized in childhood brain cancer, in the whole province, was right here in my very own backyard. She was a godsend.

When it was time to meet with her, Dr. Hunter told us that having chemotherapy at this point wouldn't be such a good idea because they had not been successful in treating low-grade brain tumours with any kinds of chemotherapy that were available then. I didn't think there was any point in going back to see her, but she wanted to keep me as her patient because she had seen the results of the MRI scans and thought there was a way to get rid of the tumour. She said if she worked together with Dr. Williams, they might be able to find a way of keeping the tumour under control or even removing the whole thing.

One thing I would do to keep busy in my hospital room was all of the physiotherapy exercises Corine gave me. Part of my daily routine was to practise all of the exercises I did with her on my own. Every morning before I got out of bed, I would do one particular exercise to strengthen my abdominal muscles. I would lie flat on my back in bed and bend my legs side by side, then push the trunk of my body up to the ceiling. I had to hold that position for ten seconds and repeat it ten times. Corine called these "bridges."

I didn't have the same equipment Corine had in her clinic to help me do some of my exercises, so I had to work around that. Instead of using the balance board, I tried to improve my balance by standing on one leg and then the other. There was a gym in the hospital, and I was sure that it had all of the equipment I needed, but it wasn't open to just anyone. Only the physiotherapists and occupational therapists had access to it.

My friends and family visited me all the time so that I wouldn't feel so alone. My grandmother came to be with me frequently, and so did the rest of my family. My uncles came with their families to play games with me, and so did some of my classmates and teachers. They came to tell me everything I was missing at school but not to worry about missing any homework. And occasionally, I had a hospital schoolteacher come to my room and review the curriculum with me. Ever since I started school, I was usually at the top of my class, so I was always open to working with the hospital teacher whenever she came to my room.

This was when Maya started making a difference in my life and in the lives of other patients who were staying in the SNU and ICU. She would come with my mom to visit me and would either sit with me or with some of the other patients. She brought Play-Doh and other toys from home to entertain everyone, and she would also sing to the kids and comfort them in her own ways. Maya was even a nurse's assistant. She would hand out towels and help the nurses sanitize the toys she had brought before they were given to all the young patients. Maya was only four years old but was thought of as a babysitter "on call" to many children in the hospital.

Dr. Williams came to discuss the tumour with me and ask about my seizures. I told him that I sometimes felt a strange feeling on the right side of my body. It seemed to start when I was taking shallow breaths. I felt it especially in my right hand and in the tips of my fingers. I also told him that I was seeing strange auras and sensing that something wasn't right during those periods. It was very tricky to explain these sensations to him, but he seemed to know what I was talking about. He said that I was probably experiencing a seizure and that I should tell the nurses if it ever happened again.

He explained that there are different types of seizures, but the most common ones are partial (focal) seizures; they only affect a small part of the brain and may have very specific symptoms. Sometimes the person experiencing the seizure can have a change in their senses, such as hearing, taste, vision or smell. There could even be changes in their mood, personality or behaviour. Confusion, hallucinations and loss of consciousness are also common side effects of partial seizures.

The bad ones are grand mal seizures, also known as tonic-clonic seizures. Grand mal seizures affect the entire brain and are considered extremely dangerous. They are marked by spasms of the entire body and complete loss of consciousness. Many people who have experienced a grand mal seizure won't have another one, but I guess since this has happened to me multiple times in my life, my case was considered "unique" by some people.

Epileptic seizures are kind of in the middle in terms of the intensity of seizures. They aren't as bad as grand mal seizures but are worse than partial ones. The effects can result in wild thrashing movements of the whole body, or they can be as mild as a brief loss of awareness. Most seizures last only a minute or two, unless they are more intense, though confusion afterwards may last longer.

Apparently, most of my previous seizures were partial ones. They were triggered by different things, such as fatigue and stress. A cold and the flu could also cause a seizure, not to mention a high fever. The nurses could tell if I was having a seizure by noticing the tremors and spasms across my body and the way my face changed. Other signs were excessive salivation and apnea. I could tell if a seizure was starting because I would have a strange sensation down my right arm. Luckily, I didn't lose full consciousness when I had these seizures and generally recovered spontaneously.

I also asked Dr. Williams a bunch of other medical questions that weren't really related to my tumour. I asked him about brain plasticity. I had heard of it at school but wasn't sure what it was. It sounded like our brains were made of plastic, though I had a hunch that wasn't what it meant. He laughed when I asked him this and explained that, no, brains aren't made of plastic. Neuroplasticity, or brain plasticity, refers to the brain's ability to change as a result of experiences throughout life. As we learn things and go through new experiences, the brain has the capacity to change or become flexible because it is absorbing new information. That was the real definition of brain plasticity.

I learned a lot about the brain and its functions thanks to Dr. Williams. The brain really can be a marvellous thing; I can see why Dr. Williams and Dr. Hunter went into the neuroscience field.

15

THE TRACHEOSTOMY

WHEN I DIDN'T have any visitors, I had a lot of free time on my hands. So I started talking to the nurses during their lunch breaks and when they were monitoring the SNU. Leslie, my primary nurse, told me that they had tried everything to solve the problem with my breathing but couldn't find a solution. She told me that when I slept, I "forgot" to breathe, but what she meant was that the message going from my brain to my lungs, telling them to breathe, was not going through while I slept and I therefore skipped breaths for longer than usual. The only way to help this was with a ventilator, which breathed for me while I slept, but that meant I would have to have a tracheostomy. She told me that if they did this, I would lose my voice and definitely have to stop eating and drinking, because I would lose my swallowing reflexes.

That's when she called in Dr. Adams, the respirologist at the hospital, to discuss how a tracheostomy worked and what extra precautions I would have to take. Dr. Adams was a well-known doctor around the world and had a lot of experience with tracheostomies. He was the best we could find for this. After he looked over my charts and saw my history of choking, he too recommended the tracheostomy.

Despite all the stress and trauma his job could cause, Dr. Adams was as laid-back as a doctor could get. He truly cared about all of his patients and wanted the best for them. He was the only doctor who talked to me like a friend and was the only one I could talk to about things other than my medical complications. We would talk about everyday life instead. He even wanted me to call him Uncle Bob when he did his rounds in the morning or if we ever met in the hospital outside of an appointment. That's what he wanted all his patients to call him so that they would feel comfortable and build a relationship with him. None of my other doctors had that kind of personality; they were all very focussed on being "doctors."

Some of the doctors took turns overseeing the SNU, and whenever it was Dr. Adams's turn, he would chill out at the doctor's station and answer any questions I had. It didn't matter whether they were about tracheostomy or just questions I had out of curiosity. I guess it is safe to say that Dr. Adams was my favourite doctor at B.C. Children's Hospital.

The first thing he told me to be wary of with the tracheostomy was suctioning. Because I would no longer have the ability to swallow properly, I could aspirate and some of the saliva I produced would go down my breathing pipe and into my lungs instead of going down my swallowing pipe and ending up in my stomach like usual. That would form secretions and mucus, so whoever was with me would have to suction it out with a suction catheter. Dr. Adams told me to ask to be suctioned whenever I could feel something in my lungs or at least every two to three hours, even if I didn't feel like I needed it. If I waited too long to be suctioned, my lungs would fill up with mucus and I could eventually drown in my own saliva. If I had a cold, I would probably have to get suctioned more often, because I would produce more saliva and become even more congested. If I was sick, the secretions would probably become yellow and green and thicker than usual, making it harder to suction them out.

In case the mucus got stuck to my lungs, we could instill some saline into my tracheostomy to loosen the mucus so that it would be easier to get rid of. Some patients with tracheostomies didn't like to get instilled, because it gave them a sensation of drowning, but I didn't mind it. I actually liked it, because I felt that it helped get my secretions out so that I could breathe easier.

I would have to make sure to clear my lungs completely before I went to sleep, because the ventilator would dry up the mucus and it would be harder to clean out my lungs the next morning. If the secretions dried up and formed a plug, the ventilator would sound an alarm and wake me up. We would have to keep my airway as clear as possible, or my lungs would get infected and that would cause pneumonia or another respiratory illness. I could also experience a seizure if I didn't get suctioned regularly because the secretions would accumulate in my lungs and I therefore wouldn't get enough oxygen to my brain. Suctioning would be a crucial part of my care, because it could prevent a lot of other medical complications.

For the same reason, I had to stop eating. Aspirating food would be worse than aspirating saliva. If it was just saliva, we could easily suction it out, but we couldn't do that with food. The food would block my airway which could cause respiratory arrest.

I also had to be careful not to get any water into my tracheostomy. If any water got in, it would go straight into my lungs, so if I felt any water go into my tracheostomy while I was showering,

I would have to cough it out right away. I would have to give up swimming, because I would definitely drown within minutes if I went underwater with my tracheostomy. Swimming was one of my favourite hobbies growing up, but now it wouldn't be an option for me.

Dr. Adams said that I would have the choice of wearing one of two kinds of small caps over my tracheostomy to keep out any dust or other particles. The more common one was the HME, short for "heat and moisture exchanger," or "nose" as they called it in the hospital. It would filter the air that I inhaled and provide heat and moisture to my lungs, just like the nose on your face does. It would be easy to breathe when I had the HME on, but the downside was that I wouldn't be able to talk. Whenever I would try to talk, the air would go straight out of my tracheostomy and I therefore wouldn't have an audible voice.

The other one was known as the "speaking valve." The speaking valve would trap all of that air and force it past my vocal chords and out my mouth, making my voice a little bit louder and stronger. But the speaking valve would dry up my tracheostomy, because it didn't provide the humidity the HME did. It also wouldn't be as comfortable for me to breathe with, because I would be more used to the HME, and this would be a different way of breathing. Dr. Adams told me that I would probably only be able to tolerate the speaking valve for half an hour to forty-five minutes every time I used it. But at least I could always take breaks.

Another big concern with the tracheostomy was hygiene. Keeping the tracheostomy free of any bacteria or germs was a very important aspect of having a tracheostomy, and we had to do our best to keep it clean. We would have to keep a two-by-four gauze around the stoma and the nurses would have to change it twice a day, once in the morning when I woke up and once before I went to sleep. They would have to clean my tracheostomy stoma every day to make sure it didn't get infected. Every time anybody suctioned me, they would have to wear gloves to make sure they didn't spread any germs. They would also have to change the tracheostomy itself once a month to protect it from infection.

The ventilator was another story. It had a circuit that would attach to my tracheostomy and blow air into it. The nurses would have to change the circuit twice a week and soak it in vinegar, because it was believed that the vinegar would kill any bacteria growing in the circuit. Whenever I went to sleep, someone would have to inflate the cuff with two or three millilitres of water to prevent the air the ventilator produced from escaping through my tracheostomy stoma.

Another reason why the doctors were hesitant about doing the tracheostomy was that there were only a handful of other children in all of British Columbia with a tracheostomy and they didn't know how well it worked with children. They did so many tests on me and asked me so many questions about it that even I expected something in return for all of this.

Once I had heard all of the negative things that had to do with the tracheostomy, I begged Dr. Adams to find an alternative to solve my breathing problems. Anything but the tracheostomy. But he said they had tried everything and the tracheostomy was the only thing left. He really didn't want it to come to this, but there weren't any other solutions to choose from. Bottom line, the tracheostomy was always the doctors' last choice, partially because it was so hard on the patient and partially because of all the risks involved.

There was, however, one not-so-bad thing about having the tracheostomy, and that was that I could breathe out of it. If anyone passed gas, or if there was another kind of foul smell around me, I could ignore it and breathe out of my tracheostomy. It was just like breathing out of your mouth; you didn't have to smell the air you were breathing.

The day came when the doctors were ready to do the surgery. I was told that this would just be a quick day surgery and it wouldn't take as long as my brain surgeries. An ENT (ear, nose and throat) specialist cut open the tracheostomy stoma, and then inserted the tracheostomy Dr. Adams had picked out for me.

While I was recuperating, two of the ICU nurses started training my parents to take care of the tracheostomy and taught them what to do in case of an emergency. My parents didn't train Ashkan or Maya, but they explained everything about the tracheostomy to them and later taught them how to suction me.

I had to get used to having the tracheostomy and being on the ventilator. The respiratory therapist had to decide all of the settings for the ventilator, such as how many breaths it would take per minute and at what level it would sound the alarm.

I tried wearing the HME at first and then tried the speaking valve, but found it very uncomfortable and hard to breathe with. I couldn't talk with just the HME on, but I could when I was attached to the ventilator, because it worked in a similar way to the speaking valve, just without the discomfort. It blew air into my tracheostomy and put more pressure on it so that the airway was covered and the air that I blew would come out of my mouth instead of the tracheostomy.

The suctioning was another thing I had to get used to, and I didn't like it at first, but after a while it became routine and I didn't mind it. Whenever somebody suctioned me, they had to go down my tracheostomy with a suction catheter to a maximum depth of 9.5 cm and try to suction out the secretions in my lungs. They couldn't go any farther, or the catheter would irritate my lungs. I could feel what lobe the secretions were in, so I could direct the nurse to push on that area of my chest to get the mucus out. I had to synchronize my cough with their push so that I could cough out all of my secretions at once.

When it was time for me to go to sleep, I had to wear a Velcro strap around my chest to keep the ventilator tubing from falling over. We had to tie the trach ties in a knot around my neck to keep the attachment in place. When I first came off the ventilator in the mornings, I had to be reminded to take deep breaths over and over to make sure I was breathing independently. Every morning, when the nurses were convinced I was breathing on my own, they would suction me to make sure there was nothing left over in my lungs from the night before. They explained that the ventilator could have dried up any mucus that we missed from suctioning the night before, and those secretions could form a plug. The plug could travel to my lungs and cause pulmonary embolism, which would in turn cause respiratory arrest.

If I wasn't on the ventilator and I had a seizure, I had to be manually ventilated with an Ambu bag, a big pump that attached to my trach. Whoever was with me had to attach it and slowly pump air into my lungs until the seizure subsided. If they pumped the bag too fast, I could hyperventilate and it would cause more problems.

In the event of a power failure at night, the ventilator had a backup battery that would last a couple of hours after the original battery died. The nurses would have to make a timely decision as to where to go for an alternate power source. If a power outage occurred and the ventilator battery was dead, they would have to wake me up right away and take me off the ventilator as soon as they could, and I would have to breathe on my own.

There really were a lot of complications to be careful of with the tracheostomy, so from this point on, my family and I had to be on our tiptoes, worrying about everything that could go wrong with the tracheostomy.

16

MORE CHANGES

I CONTINUED TO GO for monthly MRIs as ordered by Dr. Williams, just to make sure the tumour was stable. After one of the scans, Dr. Williams noticed the tumour had grown slightly since the last MRI. He told me the tumour was still operable, because even though Dr. Rice had operated on it in Toronto, he didn't de-bulk much of the tumour itself. He mostly just drained the cysts in the pons of my brain, so there was still room to de-bulk the tumour further.

Dr. Williams called my parents and told them the results of the scans and that he could arrange to send me to any of the hospitals we had researched when I was first diagnosed to do another surgery, or even back to see Dr. Rice at Sick Kids Hospital. However, I discussed this with my parents and we decided that we felt comfortable with Dr. Williams and wanted him to do the surgery.

At our next appointment with him, Dr. Williams told me that if we chose to do another surgery on the tumour, I would likely lose my ability to walk. He said that I would have to use a wheelchair and that I may lose function in my arms. He called in an occupational therapist to take measurements and help me choose a wheelchair in case I needed it. Being wheelchair dependent was the last thing I wanted, so in my mind, I refused this. I even threatened to throw the chair over the Lions Gate Bridge if they gave it to me.

By then my motor skills and walking were getting worse. I could still walk by myself, but I had to be monitored at all times. Going up and down stairs was also becoming a problem. I would get tired very easily and slowly started decreasing my daily activities. I had decreased sensation to my fingertips and feet. The difficulty with my fine-motor skills prevented me from doing some everyday activities, such as fastening buttons, putting on shoes and tying laces. I always liked to play Scrabble, but I was having trouble picking out the tiles and placing them on the board. In the end we decided to do another surgery because all of my symptoms were starting to come back and they would probably get worse if we didn't do anything about it.

On the day of the surgery, I went on a stretcher into the OR, where I met with Dr. Williams and some of his colleagues. The doctors worked on me for six to seven hours and de-bulked the tumour to where my C2 vertebra had been. Once the doctors were finished operating on me, I woke up in a recovery room and was later moved into an isolation room in the ICU.

The doctors sent a sample of the tumour to Texas for a pathology assessment to analyze the tumour. They found that the pathology of the tumour had changed, and although the tumour was not malignant, it was expected to regrow.

Following surgery, I remained bed-bound and quite weak but gradually gained strength over the next few weeks. By three weeks post-surgery, I was beginning to stand and take small steps with the help of my nurses, something Dr. Williams didn't think I'd be able to do again.

But not everything came out perfectly after that surgery. I started having spasms and tremors in my right leg. My mom talked to Corine about this and she said that the best way to get rid of a spasm in my leg was to simply bend it or lift it off the floor for a split second. If this didn't work, I could try to raise it higher off the floor, or I would just have to wait until the spasm finished.

Another result of that surgery was the weakness on the right side of my body got even worse. I was always right-handed, but now I couldn't even hold my hand up to write. I now had to type everything on the computer instead of writing with a pen or pencil. My right leg was so weak that I couldn't stand up immediately after the surgery. This took a lot of effort, but it slowly improved, even though I still didn't have the strength that I used to. I knew that I could overcome my standing problem as long as I worked as hard as I could. All I had to do was set my goal and try my best to get to it.

Another side effect from this surgery was that as soon as I woke up from the anesthetic, I started seeing double. When I opened my eyes, I saw two of everything around me in the hospital. I tried opening and closing my eyes, but it didn't help. Then I tried keeping one eye closed and the other open, and that seemed to make a difference. I thought this was just temporary, but the double vision never changed. This was hard for me to adjust to at first, especially when I was reading, but I eventually got used to it. I decided to wear a patch over one lens of my glasses so that the double vision wouldn't bother me as much.

I continued to eat solid food with limitations, but I had to be suctioned much more frequently whenever I ate, to prevent food from going into my lungs. I had to have all liquids through my G-tube, and all my medications were crushed and diluted with water, then pushed through my G-tube with a syringe. I began to think that I wouldn't have to stop eating food, even with a tracheostomy, but the nurses told me not to get my hopes up: I would definitely have to stop eating sooner or later.

I couldn't deny the fact much longer that I would have to stop eating and drinking for the rest of my life. I knew I would miss eating, especially my grandmother's lasagna; that was always my favourite meal. Dr. Adams knew this would be hard to adjust to but said that I would eventually get used to not eating. He said that I could, however, occasionally suck on hard candy and then spit out my saliva, just to get some flavour into my mouth. But even this was dangerous. If I swallowed any of the candy, it could get into my lungs and result in pneumonia.

One of the other ICU doctors inserted a G-tube into my stomach on January 19, 2001. The G-tube stoma and the skin around it had to be cleaned every day to prevent irritation of the skin and infection. Discharge from the tube was one of the symptoms of infection. So was stoma redness, heat and swollenness, or even a bad smell coming from the G-tube stoma. The nurses had to clean around the stoma with mild soap and water at least once a day. They had to dry it by patting the site, because rubbing it too hard would also cause infection or skin breakdown.

G-tubes are sometimes pulled accidentally or become blocked and need to be replaced, so when we had to change the G-tube, the nurses had to deflate the balloon and quickly pull out the G-tube. They would then insert a new one and re-inflate the balloon to keep it in place.

We had an appointment with a nutritionist to determine the right amount of nutrition. The nurses had to mix 250 cc of water with one cartridge of feed for me and pour it into a feeding bag. They attached it to my G-tube and ran the feed by gravity, with the other end hanging from an IV pole above my head. In case the feed was going too fast or too slow, I could always adjust the speed by turning the knob up or down and it would show how fast the feed was going. We had to do this four times a day: once at eight in the morning, again at noon, then at four p.m., and finally at eight in the evening.

I always had a positive attitude as a kid, and never wanted to be unhappy or negative about anything, so I tried to look at the bright side of this; at least, if I had to stop eating, my mom didn't have to spend any money buying me groceries or cooking for me. That was another reason for my childhood success: my positive attitude. I was always a happy and high-spirited person, no matter what the circumstances, and that helped a lot with everything I was going through over my lifetime.

It was very hard for me to face such adversity at my age. I was only eleven years old when all this was going on, but with all these changes I had to adapt to, I felt as though I were a full-grown adult who had endured so many hardships over his entire lifetime. When I was ready to leave the hospital for good, the nurses brought the wheelchair for me to get into the car with, but I refused to use it and said, "I'm going to walk out of this place if it's the last thing I do." And to everybody's astonishment, that's what I did.

17

CANUCK PLACE

I WAS DISCHARGED FROM the hospital in mid-February 2001 and was admitted to Canuck Place, a hospice for children with life-threatening illnesses, funded in part by the Vancouver Canucks. Canuck Place was originally a mansion that was donated by a very generous couple and renovated to become a hospice for children who were in positions similar to mine.

Not everybody got to stay there: only kids who were expected to be at the end of their lives or who were in need of a place to transition between the hospital and home. This was my first time going to Canuck Place, so I didn't really know what to expect from it, but I had heard great things about it from the nurses and doctors at the hospital. Just like some of the other kids who were staying there, I wasn't going to go straight home.

Everybody really was very caring there. The nurses and care aides made sure I was always comfortable by sitting in a big leather reclining couch and by having a bell by my side in case I needed anything. I was still having trouble with my walking, but some of the staff helped me improve it every day. Every morning I would do the physiotherapy exercises Corine had told me to do, and I would walk around the hallways and try to go up and down the stairs a few times a day, until I couldn't do any more. Two of the care aides who worked there would walk with me for especially long periods of time. I had told them my plans for the wheelchair, that I wanted to throw it over the bridge, so they knew how much I wanted to keep walking.

Occasionally we went on outings as a group, either to a park or to the movies and sometimes, if we were really lucky, to a Canucks game. The two care aides that helped me walk were usually the dedicated drivers who took us to and from the various outings. When we had the opportunity to go to General Motors Place (currently Rogers Arena), we would all be invited to watch the game from Marcus Naslund's private suite. He always donated many tickets to Canuck Place. The suite was big enough for the wheelchairs we needed to accommodate, and had leather couches and big-screen TVs on the walls. I didn't want to watch the games on a TV, so I sat on one of the stools in the suite and watched it live. We all had great views of the arena from the suite and had the time of our lives.

Another outing was to Grouse Mountain. One of the highest peaks in Vancouver, Grouse Mountain is thought of as the city's most-visited tourist attraction, receiving over a million visitors each year. I was familiar with the area, but had never been to the top of the mountain before. They had two orphaned grizzly bear cubs locked up for us to see and take pictures of. There were also a few wolves behind an electrified gate, which we were told not to get close to, because it was very sensitive and would easily electrify us intensely. The only thing I didn't like about that outing was that we didn't get to see the famous lumberjack show, which they only had during the summer.

At Canuck Place there were always volunteers who came to play games with the kids in a recreational room upstairs.

We would play countless games of Scrabble, and I usually won those games despite being five or ten years younger than all the volunteers. The Scrabble games really helped with my coordination, and we would sometimes play with the Scrabble tiles just to improve in that department.

Other volunteers would help in the kitchen. Some of the cooks were professional cooks, and some just needed volunteer hours. Even though I was not able to eat, I would still go downstairs to the dining room during lunch and dinner to interact with everyone. That was where the staff, the kids and some of the parents got together and liked to hang out, and in the end we all knew each other by name and felt more comfortable with each other.

There was a group of boys there who I would spend time with. We would play games together and just socialize. We were all about the same age, so we would also study together. It was nice to have someone my own age to relate to because the kids in the hospital were always much younger than me.

Canuck Place also had a schoolroom with a teacher who would teach us and help us with our homework. My education was always very important to me, so I worked on my school assignments with the teacher every day. She got reports from my teachers at my elementary school and was always happy to have me in her class. Having class at Canuck Place wasn't the same as going to school, but at least I knew I was not far behind everyone else with the curriculum, and that made me feel up to date. The teacher didn't only help me with my school work, but she also recommended books for me to read during my spare time because she knew I was an avid reader.

After we had a couple of hours of schooling, we would sometimes go to the arts and crafts room and have some lessons with an arts teacher. We each spelled out our names with some sort of jelly and stuck it on the window of the elevator. I didn't know how big to make it, so mine ended up being the biggest out of all of us who were currently staying in the hospice. We were told that everyone who stayed at Canuck Place did this, and their names stuck to the elevator window until they needed space for more names.

While we were in the arts and crafts room, we also got a chance to do drawings and paintings with each other. There was one girl in my class back at school who could draw like another Leonardo da Vinci, and I knew I couldn't catch up to her, so I just splattered some paint on the papers we were given and said it was the best I could do. I never liked drawing and painting anyway, so it wasn't a big deal for me.

I wasn't too interested in the music therapy program there either. I had already chosen the bands I liked, and the music therapist who came to entertain us didn't play my kind of music. I liked rock and roll, but she played soft and slow songs, so I didn't exactly like her songs. I told her how I used to play the guitar, but stopped when I was diagnosed a couple of years earlier, so I had forgotten how to play.

Staying at Canuck Place wasn't nearly as bad as staying at the hospital, but it still wasn't the same as living at home. I wanted to get back to my normal, everyday life as soon as possible.

PART TWO

A WISH COME TRUE

18

THE MAKE-A-WISH FOUNDATION

ONE DAY WHILE I was staying at Canuck Place, the nurse who was working with me told me I had a special visitor, someone I'd never met before. When the new visitor came in, she introduced herself as Jennifer Tait from the Make-A-Wish Foundation. She said that she was sent as a "wish granter" from the organization she worked for.

The Make-A-Wish Foundation is an organization that grants one wish to any child who has a life-threatening disease and isn't expected to live their full life. Since its inception in Phoenix, Arizona, in 1980, the Make-A-Wish Foundation has given hope, strength and joy to many children with life-threatening medical conditions. It is actually one of the best-known charities around the world. I knew I had outlived what the doctors had expected, and was progressing in different ways, so I wasn't going to die any day soon. I guess all that waiting in the hospital finally paid off.

First, Jennifer explained the referral process. Children who have reached the age of two and a half and are under eighteen at the time of referral, and who are diagnosed with a life-threatening medical condition by a treating physician, are eligible for a wish. Then, the foundation sends one of their wish granters to learn the child's passions and interests. The wish granters connect with the children and help explore their imaginations to determine the perfect wish. They encourage the whole family to be part of the wish experience so that they can all enjoy it together. A wish come true makes the children feel stronger and more willing and hopefully more able to battle their serious medical condition.

Jennifer wanted me to imagine everything that was special to me. Was there any special person I would like to meet? What magical place would I like to visit? What had I always wished to have? I told her my number one interest was anything to do with hockey. I already knew a lot about it, and maybe if I didn't know about Canuck Place, I would have decided right away to meet the Vancouver Canucks. But I knew that they visited once in a while, so put that idea out of my mind. I thought about meeting one of the superstars or even Wayne Gretzky, the all-time leader in the NHL with the most goals, assists and points. Gretzky had just retired from the NHL two years previously, but he was still my idol. Then I thought that if I met him, it would last just one day, and that would be it. He might just give me one of his jerseys and sign it, but that would pretty much be it. It would probably be the same thing if I wished to meet one of the big-name NHL players still active in the league. I wanted my wish to last at least a week, so I put meeting hockey greats in the maybe pile. I didn't end up wishing to meet Wayne Gretzky, but he still mailed me his Team Canada jersey from the 1998 Winter Olympics, and a signed picture of himself with all of the teams he played for during his NHL career.

I turned my thoughts to one of my favourite bands, The Police, and I thought I could do something with them. They had broken up a long time ago, but I wondered if I could get them back together for such a special occasion. I wondered if I could get backstage tickets to one of their concerts and meet the whole group. Jennifer told me that she could arrange for anything to happen with them as long as they were okay with it, so I could think of any random idea and she would try to make it happen. Maybe I could have an entire venue to myself and my family and they could have some sort of concert just for us. Maybe Sting could even sign my guitar!

If that didn't work then I also thought of doing a similar thing with The Guess Who. I knew how famous they were, and thought that meeting them would be a real honour. Ever since I was a little kid, I preferred older music from the '70s and '80s to the music I grew up with in the '90s and '00s. I imagined learning to play some of their songs on my guitar and doing my best impression of "American Woman" for them and seeing how they rated it. But we already had some of their albums at home, and I thought that I could think of better opportunities for my special wish, so I also put that in the maybe pile.

The 2002 Winter Olympics were coming up the following year in Salt Lake City, Utah. I had never seen any Olympic events live before, and here was my best chance to fulfill that dream. I thought maybe I could ask for tickets to the men's hockey tournament and maybe even give out the medals! That way I could meet all of the best players who were chosen to compete in the Olympics, and it would be some kind of vacation at the same time. That would be like a two-in-one. I could also go to some of the other events, and go with my whole family. I didn't know the entire roster for the hockey tournament yet, but I was sure it would be full of superstars. I got very excited about this idea. This sounded like the perfect wish to me, but this was only the first day that I was going through my options and I didn't want to jump to conclusions.

I asked Jennifer to give me some ideas to choose from and she told me about some of the previous wishes that had been granted. She said that some children wish for a room makeover of something that they really like and can never get enough of. Some children wish for the latest and greatest TV or laptop or some other kind of electronic device. Some of the kids they helped wished to go on vacation. The most popular choice was a vacation to Disney World. Almost 50 percent of the wishes the Make-A-Wish Foundation granted were to fly to Disney World. Meeting a celebrity or somebody famous was also a wish commonly granted, but I had already thought of that.

I imagined having an NHL room makeover, but guessed it would just be a couple of paintings and posters of players on the walls, and decided I didn't want to waste my wish on that. I told this to Jennifer and she told me that it didn't have to be just posters and pictures. They could bring in professional designers and I could customize my room any way I wanted.

Jennifer suggested that I take my time and talk to my family about this because there were a whole lot of different things I could choose from and I needed some advice. I needed to slow down and think it all through.

19

BRAINSTORMING IDEAS

A COUPLE OF MONTHS after I was admitted to Canuck Place, my parents came with Ashkan and Maya to pick me up and take me home. I was finally going home for the first time after so many months of being away from my friends and family. It was the last week of April and the sun was shining brightly as we packed my bags and drove home. When I first got home, Spunky kept barking and growling at me because he didn't recognize me, but once he got used to me, he became my best friend. He would follow me everywhere and always sit by my side. Every day Spunky would jump up on my legs and I would start petting his head. I would continue to pet him and scratch the back of his neck, and he always thoroughly enjoyed it. He would moan and groan and really sink himself into my hand until he had had enough of my love. Maybe he could sense that something was different with me because he never did this with anyone else.

After that he would just lie down on the floor beside me and not move until I did. Every time Spunky went up to anyone to be petted, there was a catch. He would jump up on my dad's lap if he wanted to be fed, he would go to Ashkan or Maya if he wanted to go for a walk, he would growl at my mom if he wanted a treat, but with me his love was unconditional. He knew that I never fed him, so he didn't growl at me when he was hungry. He only came to me for pure love and affection. Now I know why they call dogs "man's best friend."

Since I now spoke in just a whisper, I knew I had to stop answering the phone because the person on the other end of the line wouldn't be able to hear me. Whenever someone called, I would just ignore the phone until one of my family members answered it.

On my first day back at school, I thanked all my friends and teachers for their support: for the get well cards, for their visits to the hospital and for the humongous bouquet of balloons that had been waiting for me in my bedroom when I got home. While I was staying at Canuck Place, they had all chipped in to surprise me with a bouquet of flowers with a bunch of balloons attached and a big welcome-back card, in which they had all written a short note. They all wrote very encouraging messages to give me hope and strength to carry on while I was in the hospital.

I had said my last goodbyes to them when I was first admitted to the hospital, in case I never saw them again. None of us knew what was coming up or what to expect. We definitely didn't know if I would come back to school or not. But now that I was back, my classmates were all happy to welcome me back into their circle of friends.

There might have been more of a surprise amongst them when they saw me for the first time with the trach if it weren't for the video I had made with the nurses at the hospital, showing and explaining all the changes that had to be made to my lifestyle because of the tracheostomy and G-tube. While I was in the hospital recovering from the trach surgery, the hospital had also sent a couple of nurses to the school to explain why I needed the tracheostomy and how it helped me. I didn't mind my friends asking me questions about it because I knew the tracheostomy wasn't very common. I tried to answer them, but they could barely hear me because I couldn't stand wearing the speaking valve and my voice was too soft for them to hear. The nurses had to repeat everything I explained to my classmates.

Because my fine-motor skills were so bad, I needed some help writing, so the school provided me with a scribe who took notes about everything the teacher taught us. She was always very nice to me and sometimes helped me with my homework. Going to school with a nurse and having a scribe do all my writing for me definitely made me stand out, but that's what I needed. I felt like everyone else was so much more independent than I was, and that's what I wanted to succeed in the most: independence.

There was also a woman who worked at the school who specialized in brain injuries and kept coming in to see me during class. She kept insisting that I take breaks from my schoolwork and close my eyes every now and then because I was putting too much stress on my brain. I didn't want to fall behind in my class, so I didn't do this very often. She tried to modify the curriculum for me, but I always wanted to do everything everyone else was doing so that I would get the same education as my classmates.

I kept working on my balance with Corine because I didn't want to use the wheelchair the hospital had given me. When I came home from school, I tried to just hold onto the rails of the stairs and walk up the stairs. Walking on flat floors wasn't bad, but going up and down stairs was more of a challenge. I had a few episodes of tripping over my own feet when I was walking down the stairs at home, but at least the school was all on one level, so I got to take a break from the stairs while I was there.

My friends and their parents would invite some of us to their homes for pizza and movie nights and I would sometimes go with my parents or nurses. Even though I was still getting accustomed to all the changes that had happened over the past year, I still wanted to fit in with everyone else. My nurses and parents compromised by giving me some time alone with my friends but staying close enough just in case I needed them.

Now that I had a tracheostomy and didn't have any swallowing reflexes, I couldn't eat anything, but I still sat with everybody at mealtimes and we all shared stories of our lives. I always considered myself one of them even though I was, in some ways, different than everyone else. None of my friends had to be monitored 24/7; they could all eat and drink whatever and whenever they wanted; they were all fully mobile; none of them had to worry about a tracheostomy or a G-tube; and I'm sure none of them had double vision.

I told them about the Make-A-Wish Foundation and that they would grant me one special wish. My friends gave me some good suggestions for wishes I hadn't thought of. Some sounded pretty good and some I wasn't too interested in. We went through all the pros and cons of their ideas, and I finally decided that I wanted to go on a vacation for my wish. I would go away for at least a week and my whole family would come with me. We would have to carry a lot of supplies around with me now that I had a tracheostomy and needed a ventilator, but we had the Make-A-Wish Foundation to help with that.

This was my chance to go anywhere in the world. I felt like I really had to take advantage of this opportunity. I wanted to go somewhere far away, somewhere unique that wasn't like an everyday vacation. Places like New York or Hawaii were too common. I wanted to experience another culture and scenery other than what we were used to in Vancouver, so I set my thoughts on any continent other than North America.

I was most keen on going to Europe instead of any other continent because I was interested in old architecture and I knew there was a lot of history there. I had already visited one of the Seven Wonders of the Modern World when I went to see the CN Tower in Toronto, and when I thought about the other ones, the Eiffel Tower in Paris came to mind. Maybe that wasn't one of the wonders of the world, but it still interested me. We all spoke French except for my dad, so going to France was a possibility. The problem with Paris was that it was too modern. It was probably like another Vancouver, but without all the scenery we had in British Columbia.

I hadn't decided on what exactly to do for my special wish yet, but at least I had narrowed down my options to going on a family vacation.

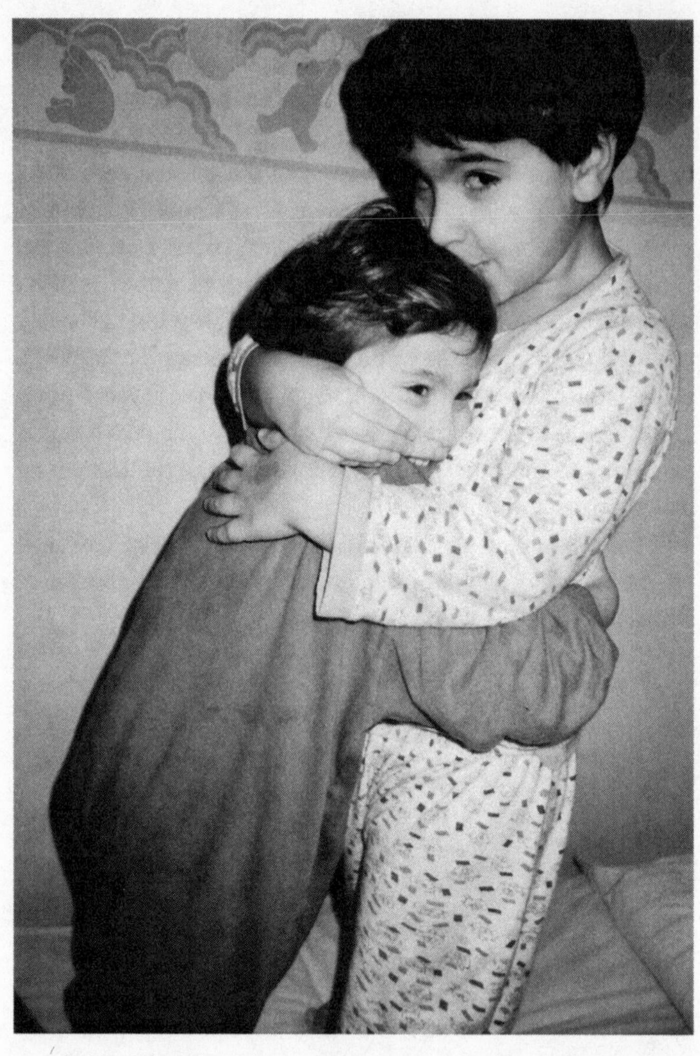

One of many special moments with Ashkan in our childhood days, in 1993.

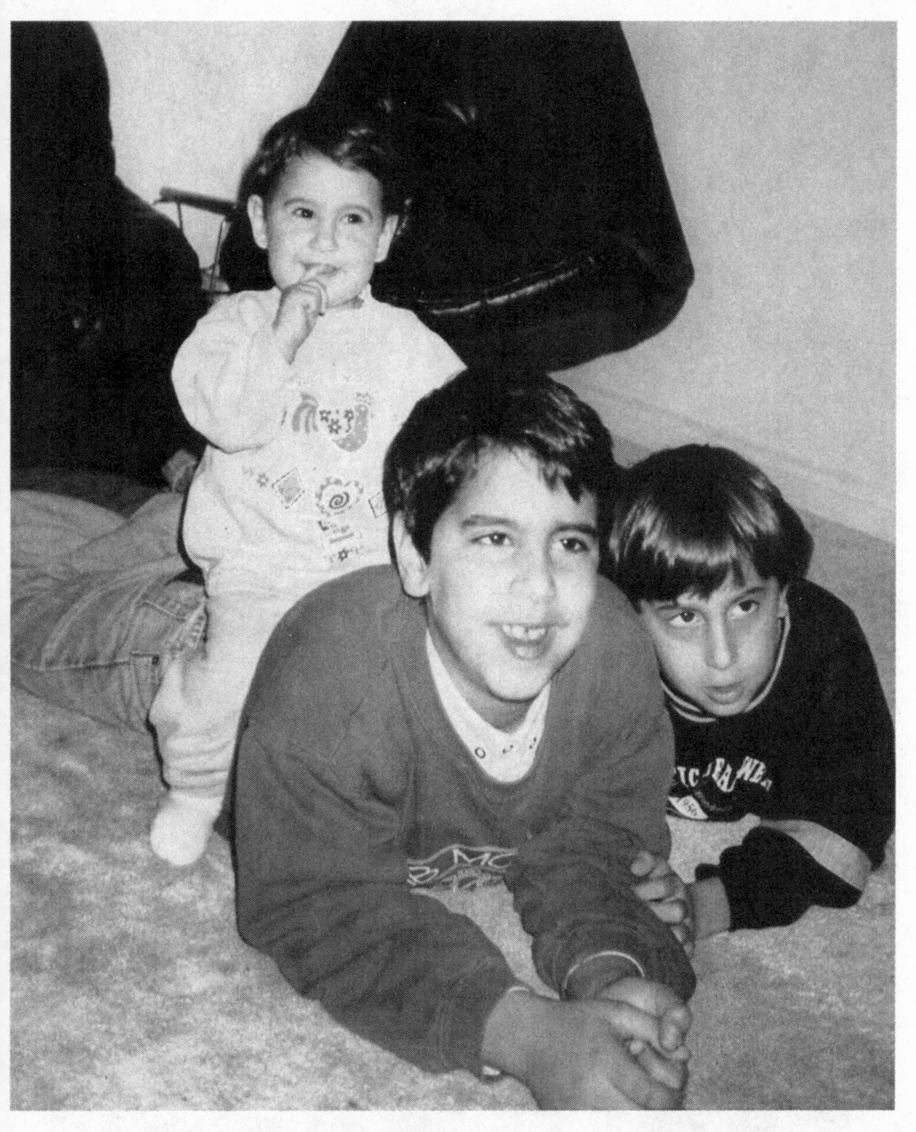

From left to right: Maya (10 months old), Bayan (6) and Ashkan (4), in 1995.

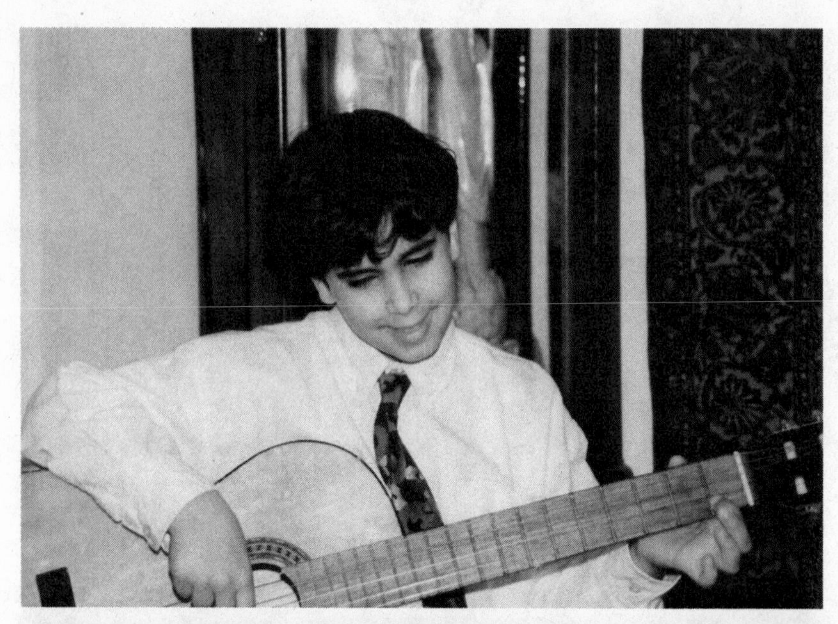

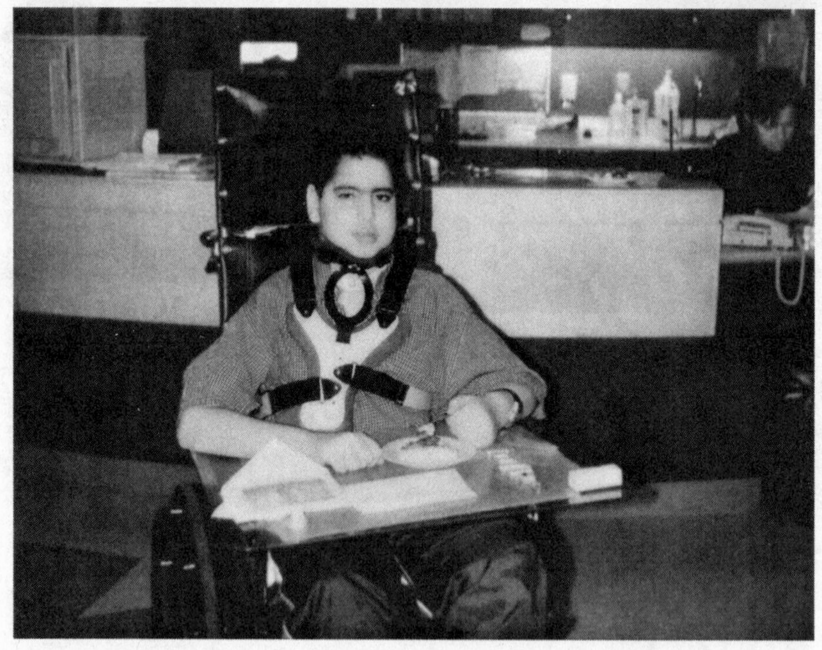

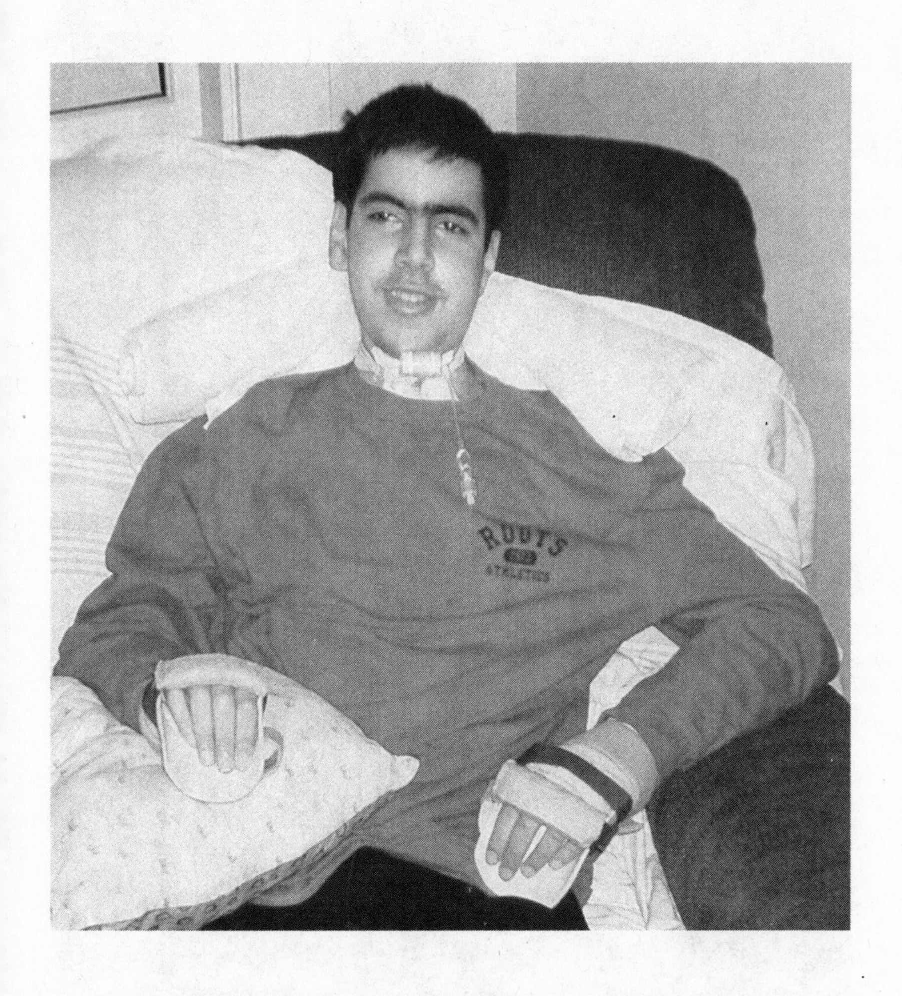

FACING TOP: Playing my guitar at Grandma's house on my birthday in 1998, before my diagnosis.

FACING BOTTOM: Recovering from my second surgery at B.C. Children's Hospital in 2001. I was still able to eat solid foods then.

ABOVE: My special "throne" at Canuck Place, in 2005, just after my last surgery.

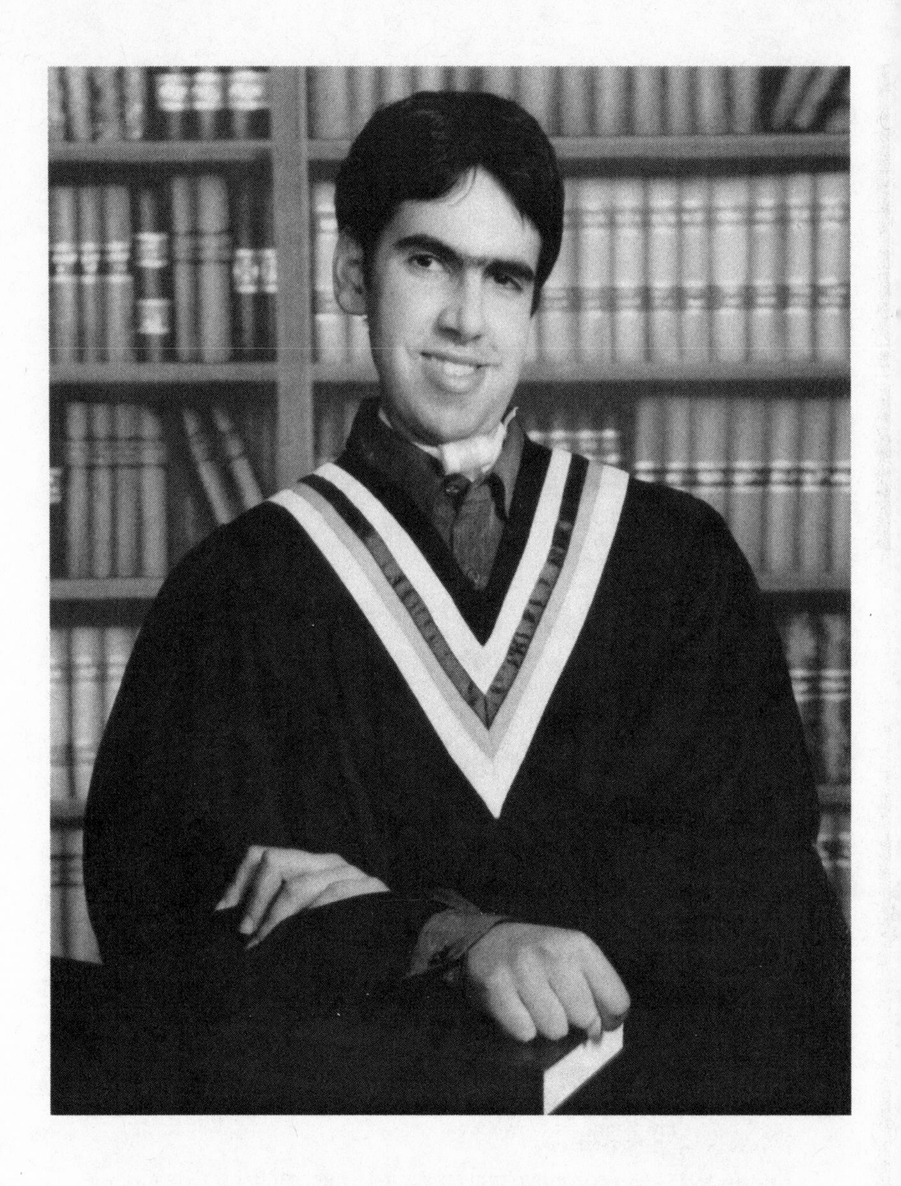

ABOVE: My graduation photo, from the Argyle Secondary School graduating class of 2007.

FACING TOP: On one of my kayaking adventures in Deep Cove in 2013.

FACING BOTTOM: My mom and me on a hiking trail in West Vancouver in 2013.

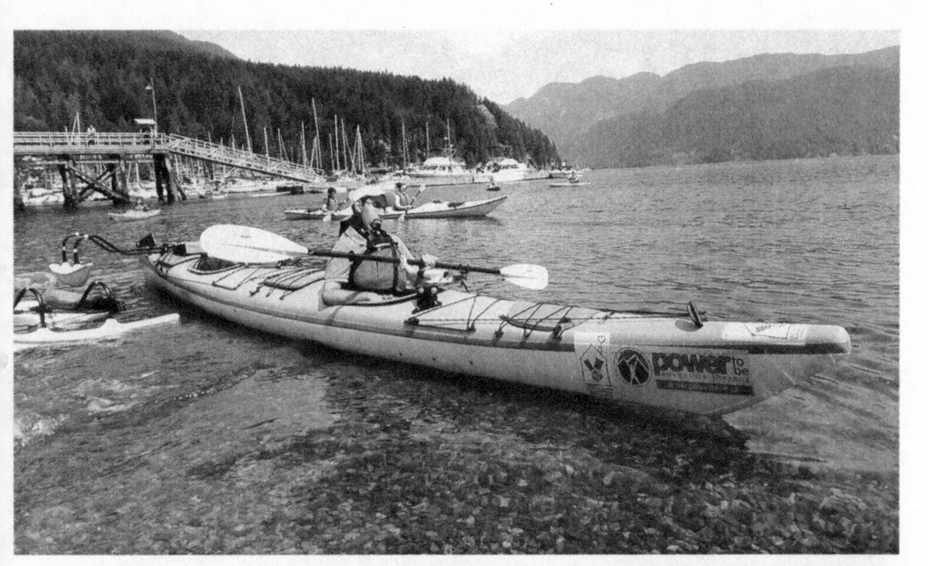
power to be

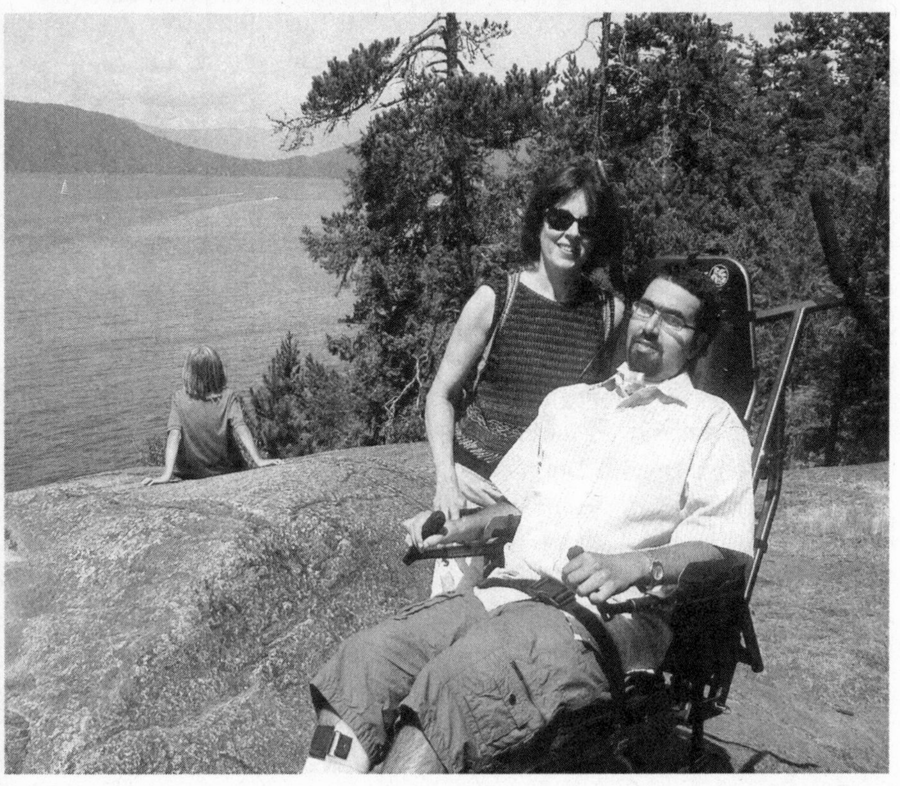

20

CANUCK FEVER

ONE DAY IN October, my mom got a phone call from the recreational therapist at Canuck Place telling her that I was invited to return for the annual pumpkin carving taking place in a few weeks. Every year at the end of October, the Vancouver Canucks come to visit the kids there and carve pumpkins for Halloween. I got all excited about this and immediately gathered the merchandise I had at home for the players to sign. I thought about wearing my Brad May jersey, but knew it was too big for me, so I just packed it in the car to bring with us.

When we got there, I sat down at a table in the kitchen with Ed Jovanovski, one of the Canucks' defencemen and alternate captains. His wife had come with him and she was standing at our table, right behind us. She had long brown hair tied back into a ponytail and was wearing a big diamond ring on her left ring finger. A bunch of the other players and their families were carving pumpkins with the other kids. Maya and Ashkan were sitting at another table in the kitchen with Dan Cloutier, the Canucks' starting goalie.

After we introduced ourselves Jovanovski asked me what pattern I wanted to carve into the pumpkin or if I just wanted to carve a normal jack-o'-lantern. I had never carved a pumpkin before, so I didn't even know how to do it. I just wanted his autograph on one of the pucks I had brought from home. I looked around at the other players and wondered if I could get their autographs too.

Somehow Jovanovski and I began talking about the attacks on the World Trade Center, a.k.a. 9/11, which had just happened in New York less than two months previously. It was big news all over the world, and I couldn't help but bring it up. I was still wondering about why it happened. I didn't know much about it and asked him what he thought, but he didn't think we should be talking about it, so I changed the subject back to hockey.

There were some rules I was unsure of so I asked him to clarify them for me. I asked Jovanovski which team had drafted him and in which year. Apparently, he was drafted in the 1994 NHL draft by the Florida Panthers and then was traded to the Vancouver Canucks in January 1999 as part of a seven-player trade that included Pavel Bure, one of the Canucks' star players. (When I first heard that the Canucks had traded Bure, I thought that their general manager was out of his mind. I loved watching how fast Bure skated and all the great moves he made to score, and didn't think the Canucks would ever trade him. They didn't call him the Russian Rocket for nothing.) We talked about all the inside things in the NHL. He asked me a bunch of questions, all of which I answered correctly, and he also taught me some new things. We took some pictures together, and then went back to carving the pumpkin.

Then I told him about the Make-A-Wish Foundation and how I was trying to decide on what I wanted to do for my wish. I still hadn't decided on where I wanted to travel with my family, so I asked him for some advice. I asked him where he would want to go if he had the opportunity to travel to any city in the world. He said he would need time to think about that, but it would probably be somewhere in Europe. Somewhere in France or Italy would be good. Maybe even Spain or Greece.

In the end, we didn't finish carving the pumpkin, but I was too mesmerized by sitting down with an NHL player to even care. I then went around the room, collecting players' autographs on my jersey. I had Mattias Ohlund's rookie card among the hockey cards I had collected with Ashkan, so when I got to him, I asked him to sign that too. Then he and I took pictures together and we all went upstairs and played some board games with the other kids there. After Ohlund played one game of Scrabble with Ashkan and me, my brother and I went back downstairs and played some foosball with Marcus Naslund and Trevor Linden, two of the Canucks' former captains.

We went back to Canuck Place the next day because the players volunteered to come back and spend the whole day with the kids there. Ashkan and I stayed outside with Dan Cloutier and played some basketball with him. We drew a three-point line on the ground and tried to get as many points as we could.

Then I had the idea of trying to score on him while he tended a hockey net. He was, after all, an NHL goalie, so I wanted to test myself against him. That afternoon he, Trevor Linden and I made an advertisement for the *Province* newspaper to promote the fourteenth annual Canucks for Kids Fund Telethon. Then we went inside and talked and joked for a while, and took more pictures before we all went upstairs to the games room until lunchtime.

At lunchtime I sat with everyone and explained why I couldn't eat with them. Some of them apologized for eating in front of me, but I was getting used to not eating by then and was all right with seeing others eat around me. I would always sit with my family during dinnertime at home unless there was something I wanted to watch on TV. That was usually a Canucks game.

When it was time for the players to leave, I thanked them for spending all this time with us. I never imagined spending so much time with so many famous players, but I actually got a chance to do just that, and had a great time with all of them.

21

ARGYLE SECONDARY SCHOOL

AT THE END of my last year of elementary school, my class planned a trip to Quebec City to celebrate our final days of school before the summer holidays. I had to go with my mom and one of the nurses who was taking care of me at home so they could both routinely take breaks from taking care of me.

While we were in Quebec, one of my classmates, whom I was very close to, got sick with the flu, and I spent a lot of time with him while he recovered from his illness. I told him to stay strong and be patient, just like I had to when I was recovering from my surgeries. I could relate to him being sick and having to stay in the hospital, so I could give him some hints and pointers about being bed-bound all day. We also played a lot of card games to help pass the time. He was one of the best friends I'd made in elementary school, and he had already done so much for me while I was in the hospital, so this was my chance to really show my appreciation.

When we arrived back home, he wrote me a letter to acknowledge our friendship. Here is a quotation I pulled from it: "I really want to be just like you, courageous, loving, and determined." Those words meant a lot to me and stay with me to this day.

That summer there weren't too many complications to deal with, but before September I had to decide whether I wanted to stay in French immersion for high school, or if I wanted to change into the regular English program. Most of my classmates had already decided that they wanted to transfer into the English program for high school, but I still hadn't decided. My cousin, who was in my elementary class, had decided that she wanted to continue in French immersion, and she finally convinced me to go with her to Argyle Secondary School even though it was further away from the neighbourhood we lived in. There were also a few of my other classmates who were going to this school, so we weren't the only ones continuing in French immersion.

When I started high school later that year, my mom would drive my nurse and me to and from school every day, so I didn't have to worry about catching the bus. I had a daily routine that I performed every morning, including all the physiotherapy exercises Corine had given me, and I tried to finish it on time before we had to leave.

On my first day there, the school assigned a scribe from the Learning Support Centre (LSC) to work with me, just like my other aide in elementary school. Her name was Laura, and she would go with me from class to class and help write down all the information I needed. She even helped me with my homework during my LSC block. Laura told me that when she first met me, I struck her as an extremely polite person, but rather reserved; she too could tell that I liked to keep my inner thoughts to myself. She knew that I was facing an obstacle or two in my life, but I presented myself with quiet determination and a sense of strong spiritedness.

Due to my slow walking, Laura and I would leave each class five minutes earlier than everyone else so we could get to the next class before the bell went and the thousand other students in the school crowded the hallways. The nurses complained that it would be so much easier for them to walk with me if I was using the wheelchair, but I wanted to keep walking and refused to use it. I sometimes considered the wheelchair because the school was so big, but something in my mind told me to keep walking. It was hard to keep walking all day, but that determination made it possible for me to stay strong.

Mr. Inkster, one of the LSC teachers, found a private room for me to rest in with my nurses after a couple of hours of school and rushing from class to class. I used this time to lie down and close my eyes so I wouldn't tire myself out too much. Sometimes, I did the opposite. I spent my time in that room doing some physiotherapy exercises, different than the ones I did when I got out of bed in the morning. I always wanted to work hard with my physiotherapy because I wanted to maintain my strength and succeed in every way possible.

Just a couple of weeks into high school, I was in my grade eight honours math class, doing a group project, when I met another student who was just as passionate about school as I was. Her name was Allyson. Allyson introduced me to some of her friends and I introduced her to my cousin who had persuaded me to attend this school and another of my friends from elementary school who also continued in French immersion. We started socializing more and soon became friends. We talked about how I came from the other side of North Vancouver to come to Argyle, and how she lived close by and didn't have to commute far to get to school.

There was one conversation in particular we had that really stood out for me. We were talking about whether we had considered what any of us were going to do after high school, and

Allyson said that she already had some interest in doing something with kinetics—maybe becoming a physiotherapist or even an occupational therapist. This kind of excited me because I was already a little bit familiar with these two topics. I told Allyson about how I had to have my top two vertebrae removed from my spinal cord and how Dr. Robinson wanted to fuse my neck and put the rods in to stabilize it, but my neck had fused itself thanks to all the physiotherapy. I also told her about all the physiotherapy I did with Corine and offered to give her some hints about having a career in that field. I was very surprised that Allyson already had an idea of what she wanted to do as her career, for I didn't have a clue what to do after high school.

There were some days when a nurse wasn't scheduled to work with me because either their schedules were too full or the agency couldn't find anyone for my level of care, so my mom had to take their place. Not only would she drive me to school, but she would also take care of me all day, and go from class to class with Laura and me, just like the nurses would. When I was in class, she would sit with me and mostly just read books and do paperwork for home. She met Allyson and all of the LSC teachers and felt that I was in good hands at this school. They were all very supportive of me throughout high school, and it was partially their help that got me through the last five years of school.

I knew having your mom with you all day at school wasn't usual, but neither were any of my other needs, so it wasn't too hard to accept. It was then that it dawned on me that I just had to take whatever life threw at me and live with it. Everybody had given up on me long before I had started high school, but the main thing was that I hadn't given up on myself. Nobody thought I would live to even finish elementary school, especially not with my neck completely intact, but my sheer willpower and determination proved them all wrong.

22

MAKING MY DECISION

THE NEXT TIME I met with Jennifer from the Make-A-Wish Foundation was in the winter of 2002, just as the new calendar year had begun. I told her that I had decided to go on vacation in Europe, but hadn't decided which city I wanted to visit yet. We brainstormed all the popular cities in Europe and researched all their famous attractions. The Eiffel Tower was in Paris, the Colosseum and the Sistine Chapel were in Rome, many famous sculptures and structures were in Athens, the gondolas and canals were in Venice, the Leaning Tower of Pisa was in Pisa, and Belgium and Switzerland were famous for their chocolate. I wondered if there were any remains of the world wars and the Nazis in Germany. I chuckled to myself when I thought of all the historical things there were to see in Europe compared to whatever there was in Vancouver—not much except the mountains and the ocean.

Rome, Venice and Pisa were all in Italy, so going on a tour of Italy would mean I could see all of these cities. Jennifer said she might be able to arrange for that, but when she checked on it, she found out that we would only have a very short time in each city. I didn't want to be rushed during our stay in Italy, so I had to choose between the three cities. I still had Athens on my mind, so I hadn't closed the door on that, and was still considering going there.

I went home that night and discussed the dilemma with my parents. Together with my siblings, we tried to pick out all the pros and cons of each city. After that discussion, I was leaning more towards visiting Rome than Athens because of a few things. First, my mom recommended it to me because she knew that I liked Italian history and architecture, and second, I imagined that it would be easier to get around because my mom spoke Italian as her first language. My mom had been to both Rome and Athens when she was younger. She said that although there definitely was a lot of history in Athens, and I really admired ancient ruins and landmarks, they were run down and many were out in the wilderness, so wouldn't be very accessible.

There was a lot more to see in Rome, plus the attractions probably weren't as old as the ones in Athens. The glories of ancient Rome are easily accessible to anyone, mostly free, and many are in the city centre, so you can visit several places in one day. Even if we didn't have time to take an in-depth look, just walking past some of these places would be an incredible experience and give us a brief overview of ancient Rome's history. One example is the Colosseum of Rome, a huge amphitheatre that could hold up to fifty-five thousand people. I researched all the other tourist attractions in Rome with my family and finally made up my mind about my wish. I wanted to go on vacation to Rome, Italy.

The next time I saw Jennifer, I told her what my final decision was. She started looking into flights to Rome, hotel accommodations, tours and sightseeing packages and everything else we needed for our stay. She asked me when I would like to go, and for how long. I thought maybe it would be best if we went over the summer, for about a week, because we had almost three months off from school. But my mom knew I didn't like the heat, and she told me that it gets very hot in Italy in the summer, so she suggested we go during the spring break. Our school's spring break was in the middle of April, but that was the rainy season in Rome. I didn't want to spend this marvellous opportunity in the rain, so we had to find a flight that went to Rome in late April or early May.

The Make-A-Wish Foundation had to do some additional fundraising to fulfill my wish. The charity does not receive any government funding and relies solely on funds raised through donations and special events to provide wish experiences. They are able to grant wishes thanks to the support of generous individual donors, and they accept any kind of donations, from airline miles or hotel points to building supplies or computer equipment. There are golf tournaments that take place every summer to support the foundation. These tournaments have helped raise funds from all over the world.

We also had a family friend who donated a lot of money to help make my vacation possible. She and her family saw me as an inspiration and wanted to help support me in any way that they could. It was a very generous deed they did for me, so we were all very thankful for their support.

The only flaw to this wish was that I thought Maya wouldn't appreciate Italy completely. She was only six years old and I thought she was too young to really appreciate all the things there were to see, especially in the museums. Maybe even I, at the age of twelve, was too young to acknowledge the great wonders of Rome to the full extent, but at least I had the opportunity to experience something that interested me.

23
ROME AT LAST!

THE NEXT FEW months seemed to take an eternity while Jennifer confirmed everything we needed for my wish. I was starting to get really excited and was telling everybody about the trip, even my doctors. They all agreed that I made a very good decision for my wish, but they each had their concerns. Dr. Williams and Dr. Hunter worried that the elevation from the flight might cause a seizure, and Dr. Adams worried that I might fall asleep on the plane and stop breathing. Maybe they were just thinking what would happen in the worst-case scenario.

A few months after I had made my final decision about my once-in-a-lifetime opportunity, Jennifer found us a flight to Rome. It was with British Airways, one of the few airlines that flew to Italy. We were scheduled to arrive in Rome in the evening, after a stop in London. The plane tickets were generously donated by the airline. Jennifer confirmed the flights with my parents, so that part of the trip was all ready to go.

The day of our flight, my uncle drove us to the airport with his family, four hours before the flight took off. We found our way to the international departures section of the airport and found Jennifer already waiting for us with some cameramen and reporters who quickly interviewed me about the Make-A-Wish Foundation and my decision to go to Rome. I didn't say much to them, for I was too excited about leaving for Italy for the first time in my life.

I introduced Jennifer to my cousins, uncle and aunt and told her how much they had helped me and how grateful I was to have them as part of my family. We all took pictures together before it was time for us to start checking our luggage, including extra bags filled with my supplies, and scanning our passports and getting on the plane. Our cousins wished us luck with our vacation and the plane finally took off, heading to Europe.

While we were on the airplane, we all tried to stay awake by watching movies and reading books. Ashkan, Maya and I were invited to meet the pilot and the flight crew in the cockpit. There were about one million buttons and wires all around the cockpit. We took some pictures and went back to our seats before the plane landed.

The flight to London took about eight hours and the flight to Rome took about four more hours. Dr. Adams, the respirologist I was seeing at B.C. Children's Hospital, thought the flight to London would be too long, and worried that I would fall asleep during it, especially since we were flying overnight. He wanted me to take the ventilator on board in case I felt like falling asleep or felt a seizure coming on. We took the ventilator as carry-on with us, but luckily I stayed awake and didn't need it.

After we cleared customs in Rome and got all our luggage sorted out, we took a taxi to the apartment where Jennifer had arranged for us to stay. Neither of my parents was really the adventurous type, so it didn't surprise me that they wanted to take a taxi instead of finding our way around with public transit.

We had been warned not to accept a ride from just any taxi that approached us, so we called one from the airport and told the driver where to drop us off. We had to request a large minivan because when we were getting ready to leave Vancouver, we had borrowed a collapsible wheelchair from one of the hospitals in case I got too tired—the chair and all of our luggage and my supplies was too much to fit in a regular car.

I had brought a booklet with some useful Italian words and phrases if we needed it, but we just let my mom do all the talking for us, for she was the only one of us who knew how to speak Italian fluently. Besides, she liked to talk... so why not? I wasn't used to speaking Italian, so I couldn't help but laugh every time I heard the Italian accent.

When we got to the apartment we all went straight to bed because we had been awake for many hours on the planes and in the airports. We slept in until about three o'clock in the afternoon the next day, and then started unpacking our luggage and looking around our new temporary home. The apartment was decorated with an antique theme; it had neon orange couches side by side in the small living/dining area. The kitchen was roughly the size of our kitchen at home, but with stools around the table in place of chairs. There were two bedrooms in the apartment, one with a queen size bed, which I had to myself. Maya and Ashkan had to share the second bedroom with two separate tiny beds, and my mother and father slept on a pullout couch in the living room.

The apartment was on the fourth floor of the apartment building, right beside one of the many piazzas in the city. The windows looked out onto the busy street, full of cars and mopeds honking their horns and pedestrians crowding the sidewalks. There were many people driving mopeds instead of cars, and I was pleased to notice they all wore helmets. There weren't many people riding bicycles in this part of town, because it was too busy and bicycles were more common for exploring quieter streets and open spaces. I loved watching all the Ferraris and Lamborghinis pass by our apartment windows since I was such a big fan of sports cars. I could tell that we were staying in a very popular part of Rome.

Outside the apartment building, there was a wonderful outdoor market with stands that sold fresh fruit, flowers, fish and little things that a corner store might sell. There were also street vendors and caricaturists selling artwork. The cafés around the piazza were usually quite expensive, but, as we discovered, once you bought your drinks, you could sit at your table and talk for as long as you'd like. There was one café in particular, close to our apartment, where my dad liked to eat breakfast every day. He always ordered his coffee black and some scrambled eggs and bacon.

We were just within walking distance from the famous Spanish Steps and one of Rome's more popular churches. Built in the 1700s, the Spanish Steps consist of 138 steps, which I tried to go up on my own on our first day of sightseeing, but couldn't get to the top of without my parents' help. From the top, we had a great view of the whole piazza. At the foot was a beautiful fountain, the Fontana della Barcaccia. This ancient fountain is a baroque fountain, carved in the shape of a half-sunken ship with water overflowing its bow. Every time we visited this attraction, Maya, Ashkan and I all took turns splashing each other with the fresh water.

For the remainder of our first day in Rome, we allowed ourselves time to investigate the neighbourhood we were staying in, browsing the streets around the piazza and walking through the Pincio Gardens. There were many trees and majestic bunches of flowers every which way we turned in those gardens. We also passed many stores that my mom was interested in checking out. The next day we planned to start all the real exploring.

The first thing I wanted to see the next morning was the world famous Colosseum, but that was scheduled for the tour we were going to take the day after. Instead, right after breakfast, we called for a taxi to take us to the Roman Forum, in the commercial, political and religious part of the city. It is a rectangular plaza, and is surrounded by the ruins of several important ancient government buildings at the centre of the city. Many of the oldest and most important structures of the ancient city used to be located on or near the Forum, but are now torn down. Over the Forum's three-thousand-year history, many monuments have been built in Rome, rebuilt, moved, destroyed, plundered or left to fall into ruin around it, so there aren't many sculptures or monuments that are perfectly preserved.

One of the passersby told us we would get a better view from one of the hills that rose above the Forum to the south, so we climbed. There were more ruins of palaces and temples up there, but what really stood out were the area's lovely gardens, shady walks, fountains (that some people even drank from) and the beautiful view.

We continued walking, taking pictures the whole way, and ended up at the Galleria Borghese, one of Rome's most famous museums. We saw many dazzling paintings from the sixteenth century, including the *Madonna of Saint Simon* by Federico Barocci, *The Triumph of Divine Providence* by Pietro da Cortona and the *Circe* or *Melissa*, which was painted under the influence of Ariosto's poetry. The Borghese Gallery may have been relatively small, but the quality of the exhibits we saw made it worth seeing.

My mom's childhood friend, Mme Pani, lived in Rome, and we had made plans to meet her outside the museum that afternoon. My mom was already thinking of buying gifts for our family back home, so her friend recommended some shopping areas that had stores for every occasion that were also wheelchair-accessible. My mom loved to go shopping, but I argued that we hadn't come halfway around the world to shop. At least, I said that we should leave this to the evening, when we were tired, but my mom had made up her mind and was not willing to negotiate.

Mme Pani sent us in the right direction and agreed to meet up with us again later to take us to Vatican City. The first store we went to was a shoe store. There were many pairs of shoes and they were strictly for women. Shoes and boots were very expensive in Rome, especially the ones that were made of real Italian leather, but after trying on a million pairs, my mom finally decided on a pair of formal shoes for special occasions. The shoe store was on the same street as a clothing store for children, and we bought some things for my cousins at home. Rome may not have been anywhere near the same shopping league as New York, London or even Vancouver, but it had plenty of top designer stores and interesting flea markets, with grocery stores mixed in with clothing stores.

I realized it was a good thing I hadn't decided to use my wish on a trip to Paris, or we would have spent all our time window shopping. We walked the streets and took more pictures until we took another taxi back to our apartment. I fell asleep anticipating spending the next day admiring ancient history instead of Italian leather.

24

ANCIENT ROME

AT HOME I always made time in the morning to do my physiotherapy flawlessly, but this week while we were in the capital of Italy, I did my exercises quickly and wasn't paying much attention to doing them correctly, the way I was shown to. I was too excited about seeing the rest of the city to worry about my posture and everything else I did my exercises for. On this morning especially, I was rushing. Today was the day I was waiting for, the day we had booked a formal tour of ancient Rome. Jennifer booked it for us before we left Vancouver. It was supposed to be perfect for first-time visitors.

First on our list of relics was the Colosseum of Rome, once the scene of gladiatorial battles and other public events, such as bull fighting, mock sea battles, animal hunts and executions, which all involved men, women and wild animals. The Colosseum is in the middle of the city, right beside the Forum, and is considered to be one of the greatest works of Roman architecture and Roman engineering. Because we were part of a private tour, we got to skip the lineups and gained special access. We entered the magnificent monument from the rear doors and got a view of the inside from one of the top levels. Built during the rule of the Flavian dynasty, the great amphitheatre is 48.25 m high, enclosing an arena of 86 m × 54 m and a base area of six acres. The free standing structure was capable of comfortably accommodating fifty-five thousand people back in its time. It was actually originally named the "Flavian Amphitheatre" when it was first built. The name "Colosseum" was not used until the seventh century.

I was very happy with the size of the tour group, for it was so small it was almost like a personal, one-on-one tour. The others were from Canada, the United States and England. (In fact, I was sure that I remembered the British travellers and their accents from the flight from London.) We learned a lot of new things we didn't know, and all of the information the tour guide gave us was pointed directly at us. I had heard of all great things there were to see in Rome when I was a little kid in Vancouver, but never really thought I would ever experience it for myself.

The inside of the structure wasn't as spectacular looking as the outside; many of the seats and floors had been ruined due to the major fires and earthquakes the structure had to endure over the years.

We were told that the lower seating section was reserved for wealthy citizens, while the upper part was meant for less wealthy citizens. We saw Roman numerals engraved in some of the front rows; just like modern arenas, numbered seats allowed people to buy designated seats, some of which would have been made with slabs of marble. I had already been to one "Colosseum" before—the Pacific Coliseum in Vancouver—but that was just to watch a live hockey game, and it wasn't nearly the same as this.

I was very impressed with all of the patience Maya had while our tour guide was explaining all of the facts about Rome. She was only six years old when we were in Rome, but stayed quiet and happy during our whole tour. She and Ashkan helped carry the bags and push the wheelchair while we were on vacation and didn't complain about anything.

We left the Colosseum content with what we had seen and learned, and headed for one of the nearby cafés for a quick lunch with the other members of our tour group. My family took a quick look at the menu and ordered a medium-sized authentic Italian pizza topped with pepperoni and cheese. The waiter must have misunderstood the order because he brought a pizza with peppers instead of pepperoni. My dad threw some extra mushrooms on his portion of the pizza, for he always craved mushrooms. My family had a quick salad after the pizza, because in Italy it is customary to have salad after the main course, as I learned.

The tour resumed after the lunch break. Our tour guide took us up the street to the Arch of Constantine, the most recent of the three remaining imperial arches in Rome. I was interested in how many parts from older structures were reused to decorate the arch of Constantine, but overall, this monument didn't compare to the Colosseum. It was part of our tour so we had to stop and pretend to admire it as much as the Colosseum. We saw a few more monuments and then concluded our big day of sightseeing by thanking the tour guide and saying goodbye to everyone else in our tour group. Back at the apartment, I studied the map and planned what to do the next day.

We didn't have a tour scheduled the next morning, so we set out to see the Pantheon by ourselves. It was one of the buildings I had done a lot of research on before we left home. The circular building was built in AD 128 and was meant to be a temple to honour all the gods of ancient Rome. It has been continually used as a Roman Catholic church since the seventh century, which explains why it is one of the better-preserved ancient Roman sites. It was also used as another popular museum that featured mostly paintings and sculptures.

Once inside, I was impressed by the dark interior, which seemed to be made up of mostly circular and square tiles and bricks on the walls. The floors had a checkerboard pattern that contrasted with the concentric circles of the square panels in the dome, which may have contained bronze stars, rosettes, or other ornaments at one time. The inside was pretty dark because the only sources of light were from the entry door and the circular opening in the apex of the ceiling. I wondered why they didn't they have any lights and what they would do in case it rained, especially in a church, if there was an opening in the roof. One of the staff members there told me that during storms and other weather problems, a drainage system below the floor handles the rain that falls through the thirty-foot opening.

Many buildings in Western Europe that have been inspired by the Pantheon have openings such as this in their roofs. It is actually the most copied and imitated of all ancient works. This building wasn't that all that spectacular looking, if you ask me. We didn't spend too long there before moving along.

We crossed the street and continued to walk down the next street until we came across the world famous Trevi Fountain, a magnificent example of baroque art and the largest baroque fountain in Rome. It is designed to look like someone is riding a chariot in the shape of a shell, pulled by two sea horses. One of the sea horses pulls the chariot slowly, while the other stubbornly resists. They symbolize the fluctuating moods of the sea.

The tradition with this fountain is if you turn your back and toss in a coin over your shoulder, you will someday return to Rome. Approximately three thousand Euros are thrown into the fountain every day. We all wanted to come back to Rome one day, so we took turns flipping coins into the fountain. I wasn't sure if it "accepted" Canadian quarters but tossed one anyway.

After taking a few pictures beside the Trevi Fountain, we glimpsed a big palace in the distance, and out of curiosity, we started walking towards it for a closer look. We learned that this was the Quirinal Palace, the "Palazzo del Quirinale" in Italian, which is the current official residence of the President of the Italian Republic. I guess you could relate it to the White House, it being the home of the American president. It was rarely made open to the public, but on this day, fortunately, we were allowed to look around.

A massive rectangular building located on the Quirinal Hill, the tallest of Rome's seven hills, the Quirinal Palace has housed thirty popes, four kings and eleven presidents of the Italian Republic since being constructed in 1583. The palace was built on this hill because the pope wanted to find a location far away from the humidity and stench coming from the river Tiber to build a summer home for himself. He wanted a place to rest that was healthier than the Lateran Hills or the Vatican, where we were going the next day.

The gardens surrounding the palace were also astonishing. There were many sets of bushes and flowers on the Quirinal Hill that must have taken a lot of maintenance and a long time to grow, considering how well-established they were. My mom was tempted to pick a few roses here and there, but Maya just took pictures of the gardens and I convinced my mom that that was enough. We didn't want to stand too long on the President's property, so we quickly found our way off the hill and into the Piazza del Quirinale.

The piazza was packed that day with pedestrians who looked like they were just walking around and enjoying the weather. I could tell that some were visitors, for they seemed to be looking at maps and taking pictures as they walked. As we walked down the street, my parents saw a caricaturist in the distance, and wanted him to draw a picture of our family. My mom talked to him for a while, and introduced all of us, and then we posed for him for ten or fifteen minutes while he did a quick sketch of our family, standing side by side and holding hands.

25
VATICAN CITY

THE HEAT FROM the sun woke me up the next morning. For me, heat and lack of air circulation triggered seizures, and I was relatively warm under my duvet cover, so I had a quick seizure in bed that morning. I was still on the ventilator at that moment, so my parents didn't have to use the Ambu bag like they usually would, because the ventilator was still attached to my tracheostomy and it was breathing for me. When I have one of these seizures, I usually don't know what is going on, but once it subsides, I regain control of my body and become more aware of my surroundings.

My mom's friend Mme Pani wanted to take us on a tour of Vatican City specifically on a Sunday because she wanted me to see somebody very special. I had no idea who it was, but would eventually find out. At first, I thought the Vatican was just another part of Rome, but after doing a little research, I learned that Vatican City is the smallest independent state in the world in terms of population and size. It was established in 1929 and even has its own flag, but only about eight hundred people live within its borders.

Mme Pani wanted to drive us around the city, but we were going to take the wheelchair in case I got too tired to walk, and she didn't have room for a wheelchair in her car, so we ended up taking a wheelchair taxi to St. Peter's Basilica, built over the shrine of Saint Peter, Rome's first Catholic pope, and regarded as one of the holiest Catholic sites.

We entered the huge structure with much respect and marvelled at the beautiful interior. I couldn't believe that we were actually standing there. St. Peter's Basilica was known to be one of the most famous structures in the world and we were standing right in the middle of the entrance. This was actually one of the reasons why I chose to go to Rome as my wish. I was so excited to view the entire interior as soon as we passed through the entrance. There was usually a proper-dress etiquette required to enter the church, but we were just going there for a couple of hours to do some sightseeing, so we didn't need to dress up.

St. Peter's Basilica has the largest interior of any Catholic church, and its dome is among the tallest in the world. There were many random sculptures surrounding us, but the most celebrated of these was the *Pietà,* which showed Mary cradling the deceased Christ in her lap. Carved when Michelangelo was twenty-three years old, the sculpture is the artist's only signed piece of art work. There was so much detail in it that I couldn't believe how he could have carved it so perfectly.

Before we left, Mme Pani suggested that we climb to the top of the dome, so we could get the best view of the city from there. We could see our apartment building and most of the famous structures we had visited during our previous days of sightseeing.

We spent a good two to three hours admiring the rest of the basilica and then moved on to the Sistine Chapel, which is inside the Apostolic Palace, the official residence of the Pope in Vatican City. This was another sight I had been waiting to see. The Sistine Chapel was another rectangular building that was built with mostly ordinary bricks. There was nothing too spectacular to see from the outside, but the inside was a different story. I had never seen a building where the entire ceiling was painted. Of course, this ceiling was painted by Michelangelo. It was originally painted by Piermatteo Lauro de' Manfredi da Amelia, but in 1508, the Pope commissioned Michelangelo to repaint the whole thing. The walls were also painted by Michelangelo and other leading painters of the late fifteenth century, including Sandro Botticelli, Domenico Ghirlandaio and Pietro Perugino. It's also home to the renowned *Last Judgement* by Michelangelo. Thanks to the extraordinary talents of these and other great artists, the Sistine Chapel has become one of the most famous art galleries in the world. I don't think I had ever seen so many paintings at once before in my life. It felt like a real honour to be standing under such a majestic dome, admiring all the beautiful works of art it contained.

Mme Pani ushered us out to the plaza around the chapel where they had set up a big screen for that special someone Mme Pani wanted me to see. Pope John Paul the Great, the pope at the time, came out on a wheelchair and was displayed on the screen that was located beside St. Peter's Basilica. Everybody cheered for him when he came out. He gave his traditional speech and then some of the people lined up, one by one, to receive his blessings.

After he was wheeled away, we spent the rest of the day walking around Vatican City with Mme Pani and visiting some of the other museums and one of the souvenir shops. They had T-shirts, flags of Italy and of the Vatican, posters of some of the monuments, framed pictures and a bunch of other small things, none of which I was interested in. Then I noticed the books in the far left corner of the store. I wanted to do more research on the city and its sights, so I bought a book that was solely about the Sistine Chapel and one that was about the entire Vatican. There were a few paintings that I wanted to hang on the walls of my bedroom, but the paintings were too big to fit in my luggage on the plane back to Vancouver.

That day was very long, but we enjoyed every moment of it, and by the time we got back to our apartment it was past our bedtimes. I don't know about Ashkan or Maya, but that day was actually the highlight of my trip.

26
HOME SWEET HOME

THE FINAL TWO days of our vacation we spent just walking around like everyone else. By then we had seen just about all of the famous sights there were to see in Rome. My family had real Italian gelato ice cream for the first time and other Italian specialties. I didn't get to try eating the meals that everyone else ate, but at least I felt like I had paid my family back for all the help and support they had given me.

We went back to take one last picture at the Colosseum and overheard the same tour guide telling a new group of tourists the same information about the Colosseum she had given us. We noticed that they had set up bleachers and found out that Paul McCartney was performing later that evening. What a coincidence! One of the most famous people in the world was having a concert on the day we were leaving. After we got our last few glimpses of the city we headed back to our apartment to get ready to go to the airport. Our flight back home was scheduled to leave at one o'clock that afternoon, so we had to pack our bags and get all of my medical supplies ready to board the plane by eleven. We said one last goodbye to the apartment staff and our neighbours in the apartment building, and then left for the airport.

When we got to the airport, the security checked our passports and we got all our luggage onto the plane. We remembered to take the ventilator on board with us even though we didn't think I would need it. I definitely was not going to fall asleep at this time of day, but we had to follow the doctor's orders.

We took the same route home that we had taken to Rome: we stopped in England for an hour and then transferred to another flight that was headed to British Columbia. The plane touched down on the runway at the airport in Vancouver about eight hours after we had left England and eleven hours after we had left Italy. The flight was a little bit on the long side, if you ask me.

My uncle, aunt and cousins came to pick us up and drive us back home. We told them about most of the things we saw. We didn't have the pictures developed yet, so we tried to describe it all. They were keeping Spunky while we were gone, so they also brought him in the car when they came to get us. He must've been excited to see us because we couldn't stop him from barking and jumping all over us.

After we had unpacked and got settled in the next morning, we went out to get the pictures and videos developed. Exactly how many pictures we took, I don't know, but we went back home with numerous packets of pictures and four video cassette tapes. Later that day Ashkan, Maya and I started going over them with our parents and chose which ones to frame. There was no way we could frame them all, or we would have spent a fortune on picture frames alone, and there would not have been enough room in the house to display them.

We went to my grandmother's house that evening and took the video cassettes with us to show the family. They were amazed at everything we saw. After dinner, I gave my cousins the presents that we had brought back for them. We invited Jennifer over for dinner the next night and gave her the souvenir we brought back for her. I was very thankful to her for helping me choose this vacation and for making my wish come true.

I returned to classes the first full week after we got back from Rome. I kept doing my standing exercises regularly with my nurses, but I did prefer someone my own age to help me. Mr. Inkster, the LSC teacher, always encouraged peer support and knew that Allyson and I were friends, so he thought of her as a peer who could help. He asked Allyson if she could do this for me, and she agreed and kindly rearranged her schedule to fit with mine so we would have time to work together on my physiotherapy. She already had an interest in kinesiology so this turned out to be a good arrangement for both of us.

Every day during our spare blocks, Allyson and I would meet in the gym and work on the standing exercises Corine gave me. I wasn't eager to tell Allyson all about my condition just yet—it was too early in our friendship to share such personal details—but Mr. Inkster had given her a brief overview of the basics to make sure we were all on the same page. Her willingness definitely helped further our relationship. At first she didn't ask me many questions about my illness because she didn't want to invade my privacy, but over time we got closer and I opened up and shared some more information about my life.

I explained my situation to Allyson and told her how Corine wanted me to work mostly on my balance. She gave me several balancing exercises to do, including standing up and shifting my weight from one leg to another, having the person who was helping me move their hands from place to place and getting me to touch their hands.

There was also a wall in the area where we were standing that I could put my hands on and walk side to side and squat down to strengthen my thigh muscles as well. As part of my physiotherapy, I had to make sure I was lifting my right leg all the way off the floor from my knee, and wasn't dragging it as I was walking. Whenever I sat down, I had to focus on sitting slowly and with control, or the fast fall would send shocks and spasms up my back. Following my return from our big family vacation, it was my priority to re-establish my physiotherapy routine.

27
COPS FOR CANCER

I WAS HAVING A lot of seizures that summer, so as an extra precaution, I stayed home most days, playing games and having fun with my nurses. My parents and nurses didn't want to risk having to manually ventilate me with the Ambu bag, so they encouraged me to stay home while everyone else, including Ashkan and Maya, was spending their days outside with their friends and stuffing themselves with ice cream. I wanted to spend just as much time outside, but my seizures were affecting me too much.

One day while I was playing a board game, one of our family friends, who was very engaged in fundraising, called my mom and told her about another charity we didn't know about. This one was called "Cops for Cancer." It is a charitable program administered by the Canadian Cancer Society and is made up of police officers who are devoted to children suffering from medical, physical or traumatic issues. They have many events throughout the year to raise awareness for children who live in the communities that they serve, and they are very successful with all of them. Their main event in the Greater Vancouver Region is the Tour de Coast, a two-week event during which they ride their bikes all over the coastal region of British Columbia and raise funds as they go.

A friend of my mom's friend was a police officer taking part in this event that year, and he was looking for a kid to ride for. He served in North and West Vancouver, so I was the perfect match for him. I wanted to meet him, so my mom set it up. When that day came, the police officer drove to our house in his own car. I was expecting him to come in his police car, but I guess he only used that when he was on duty. He introduced himself to me as Fred Harding. Fred was a tall British man with short, cropped black hair. His big smile and piercing brown eyes showed some inner warmth to me. My mom joined us and we all sat down at the kitchen table for tea.

Fred told me that the annual Tour de Coast ride was coming up and he was riding in it. This exhausting ride occurs each September, and the riders were expected to ride over some very challenging terrain. Some roads weren't even paved. Each competitor had his or her own reason for taking part and motivation to set a fundraising goal. All money raised from this event is used for life-saving childhood cancer research.

He told us that the first Cops for Cancer program started in 1994, in Edmonton, when a police officer with a shaved head posed for a picture with a young cancer patient. Since then, many police officers and sometimes entire divisions have participated in Cops for Cancer's traditional fundraising events. Through all of their activities, police officers and generous communities have helped raise over $50.4 million for cancer research through Cops for Cancer. Once Fred had finished he got up to leave. I quickly ran after him and gave him a big hug at the front door and wished him luck on his upcoming journey.

About a month later, when the ride was scheduled to start, we all drove to the starting point of the ride and met the competitors there. Two big trucks filled with food and toiletries were parked by the starting line in the plaza parking lot. One of the trucks was going to lead the way, and the other was going to follow the last rider. There was a crowd of over one hundred people surrounding the cyclists, who were ready to start their trek. They all had big mountain bikes with them, with pictures of their mentors on the bikes. Fred had taken a picture with me earlier and he now had it taped on the frame of his bicycle. There was a brief luncheon and then the starter's horn blew and the bikers all started towards the mountains for the beginning of the event.

"What a wonderful charity," my mom said, as we said goodbye to everybody and drove back home. She always acknowledged how much everyone supported me.

During the Cops for Cancer ride, while the officers were struggling to ride their bicycles along the unpaved roads, Jennifer started a competition of her own. She climbed to the top of Mount Kilimanjaro in honour of me. At the peak of the mountain she taped my picture to one of her poles. After she got back to Vancouver, Jennifer sent me a picture of herself standing at the top of the volcanic mountain, dressed in a thick winter coat and toque, which I still have framed in my room. Standing at 19,341 feet above sea level, Mount Kilimanjaro is the world's highest free-standing mountain and Africa's highest point. She climbed it to raise money for the Make-A-Wish Foundation, and was very successful in doing so.

The Tour de Coast finished just days after Jennifer gave me the picture of her standing at the top of Mount Kilimanjaro. The bikers finished their ride in front of my high school to celebrate with the students and staff and to honour me. They closed the roads to the public so they could park their bikes on the street. The whole school came outside and cheered as the police officers introduced themselves and high-fived all the students.

Fred presented me with the jersey he wore during the ride. It was bright red with the words Tour de Coast written across it in yellow ink. All the sponsors were listed in blue on the back of the sweater. It was very reassuring to know there were so many people willing to dedicate themselves to such an important cause. I hope to one day be able to make a difference in my own way.

PART THREE

WHEN THE GOING GETS TOUGH, THE TOUGH GET GOING

28
MORE SIGNS

BY SEPTEMBER WE were starting to notice some changes in my daily routine. I was feeling a lot weaker than usual and couldn't do as much physical activity as before. When I got up in the morning, I would just point to my closet or dresser and let my nurses pick out my clothes for me instead of getting them myself. I wouldn't use my right arm anymore because it was too weak to hold anything up. I would just let it dangle beside me while I did everything with my left arm. I knew my physiotherapists wanted me to use it more to strengthen it, but I had given up on my arm.

Even my walking was getting worse and going up and down stairs was becoming more troublesome. I wanted to keep walking, especially at school where everyone else was mobile, but the nurses said that it would be a lot easier if I just sat in the wheelchair and they pushed me. I agreed that it would be easier for both them and me if I just sat in the wheelchair.

I was still doing my standing and walking exercises in the gym with Allyson during my spare block, but even she was convinced that something was different. We started meeting only every other day because I didn't want to strain myself too much. Squatting was the hardest exercise for me to do precisely, so I just stopped doing the squats altogether. I told my parents and nurses I was just getting lazy, but they were sure it was something more serious than that.

My next doctor's appointment was with Dr. Hunter, the neuro-oncologist at Children's Hospital. Before my mom and I left the house, we made a list of things we wanted to address with my doctor. The increase in seizures was first on the list, but Dr. Hunter didn't want to increase my medication, so she started to wean me off my current seizure medication and tried a new one that had just come onto the market and seemed to be more effective in some cases. Since it was not clear why my seizure activity had increased she suggested that I take it easy and try not to stress myself. I agreed to use the wheelchair more frequently so that I would not strain myself.

We told her that I had already decreased my physical activity, that my school workload had been modified, and that I was taking daily rests when I got back from school, so she just wanted us to continue with that and see how it went. While we were still on the subject of not doing as much daily physical activity, we told her how I was feeling weaker and was starting to cut corners. She had a simple solution for that: just do what I could and let my parents and nurses take care of the rest.

I tried the new drugs for a while but to no avail. My mom made another appointment with Dr. Hunter and told her that nothing had changed. Then the doctor had the idea of putting me on chemotherapy to try to kill the bad cells in my brain. I had already tried one round of chemotherapy three or four years previously, while I was recovering from the tracheostomy surgery, and that one did not make much difference, so Dr. Hunter wanted to try a different kind of chemotherapy.

Because we couldn't take the chemotherapy home and give it to me like all my other medicines, I had to go back and forth to the hospital once a week with one of my parents so the nurses at the hospital could give me the treatment intravenously. It was mid-November by then, so the sun was going down earlier and the days were starting to get shorter.

The nurse had to dress up in a gown and wear a mask and gloves, and then start a small IV in the back of my hand. We kept doing this once a week for about a month, but Dr. Hunter was not noticing any benefits. Just like the last time I'd had chemotherapy, I didn't experience any of the usual side effects of chemotherapy like hair loss and nausea. Some of the other side effects can include vomiting, diarrhea, constipation and soreness of the mouth. I was, however, heavily drugged and wasn't my usual self while I was getting the treatment. I was having mood swings and felt much weaker than before we started the treatment.

Dr. Hunter didn't know what else to do except get Dr. Williams involved. She brought him up to date on the change of medication, the chemotherapy and everything my parents had mentioned, and he suggested doing another MRI to check if the tumour had changed in any way.

I got up the next morning and got ready for an emergency MRI. I got in the car with my mother and father, and drove to the hospital for my appointment with Dr. Williams. It took one hour for the MRI scans to finish, and once Dr. Williams reviewed them, he called us into his office. He told us that the tumour had changed slightly and was putting more pressure on my brain. That could be the reason for my symptoms. He said he could take a chance and operate on it again because there was still room to de-bulk it; however, this time the risk of losing more of my body function would be greater.

This time the final decision of whether I wanted to have another brain surgery was left up to me, and the doctors did not ask for my parents' input. I couldn't make that decision right there and then, so we went back home to have a family discussion. We all knew that things were getting worse, and we didn't expect them to get any better by themselves. I had tried different medicines and chemotherapies, but none of that helped. When we were discussing the possibility of another surgery with Dr. Williams, he mentioned there could be more side effects and I might need the wheelchair full-time.

I already needed the tracheostomy and ventilator, and I already had weakness on the right side of my body, not to mention the double vision I'd had to put up with since the second brain surgery, so I didn't know what else could go wrong with me. We all knew that things were getting worse and that the doctors had tried desperately to solve the problem but couldn't, so we were kind of at a dead end.

The next time we saw Dr. Williams, he strongly encouraged me to have the surgery. He thought everything would just get worse from here and I would eventually end up bed-bound if we did nothing. I was in his office with my parents when he said this, and I was sure he was right about it, so I finally gave him the thumbs-up to do my third brain surgery. No doctor likes to lose a patient, and this was probably going to be one of the riskiest operations Dr. Williams would perform in his entire career, so I was sure he would do the best he could. I knew that Dr. Williams was one of the best neurosurgeons we could get, and he had already operated on me twice before, and I therefore had a lot of faith in him.

The surgery was scheduled for December 8,2004, exactly the day of my fifteenth birthday. The doctors didn't need to explain how to prepare for surgery; I had already gone through this procedure a few times before. It was another one of those "been there, done that" situations.

I had never seen a brain tumour, except for seeing it on the MRI pictures, and was curious as to what the real thing looked like, so I asked Dr. Williams for a sample of the tumour once he removed however much he could. He said that none of his previous patients had asked for this, but he would be happy to give me part of the tumour after the surgery, as long as I didn't take it out of the bottle he would give it to me in.

I remember lying there by myself in the hospital bed, waiting for the doctors to get ready to start the surgery and thinking to myself: "So this is what I get for my birthday—another brain surgery that could mess up my life even more. Just what I need." I don't think I'll ever forget that thought.

29

MAJOR CHANGES

I STAYED IN THE Special Needs Unit until it was time for my surgery. While the doctors were working on me, my parents waited patiently in the waiting room with thoughts of despair on their minds. They and the rest of my family were worried to death that this would be the last time they would see me alive. They were praying that they hadn't just said their last goodbyes to me and that I'd make it past this surgery just like I had with the other ones. But this was the most intense and dangerous surgery that I'd had to endure so far and was probably my last chance to have a surgery, because the doctors could only go so far into my brain stem.

There was, however, one positive thing. An incredible new technology had just become available that would alert the doctors if they got too close to a nerve and prevent them from causing damage. It had taken some time for the doctors and technicians to master how it worked, which was why they'd had to postpone the surgery to the day of my birthday. I was actually the first patient at B.C. Children's Hospital on whom they were going to use it.

Everybody was surprised when I opened my eyes in my recovery room in the ICU after eight gruelling hours of intense surgery—Dr. Williams most of all. Together with the other surgeons, he had done a beautiful job removing most of the remaining parts of the tumour. He came into my room and asked me to wiggle my fingers and toes, told me to follow his finger with my eyes and did some other simple tests like asking me if I knew where I was and what day of the week it was.

A few days after the surgery, he asked if I noticed any physical changes since the surgery. I told him that I had tried standing, but couldn't without the support of two of the ICU nurses. My right leg had gone limp now, but that was precisely what Dr. Williams was expecting. He didn't think it would be my left leg because the right side of my body was the affected side. There was also a big difference in my arm. It had lost all mobility. Before, it was just weak, but now the mobility was next to nothing. I wanted to chop it off, or at least put it in a sling, but that would've caused more problems by throwing me off balance even more.

I did notice a slight change in the left side of my upper body: I couldn't feel anything when the nurses touched my arm. I could still feel that I had my arm, but I couldn't feel it when someone pinched it or poked it. The nurses wanted to see how far across my body the lack of sensation went, so they got an ice pack and held it on the outside of my chest and moved it further to the middle until I could feel it.

Even Dr. Hunter wanted to see for herself how severe the loss of sensation was. I remember her coming into my room and poking me with a toothpick to see what parts of my body were affected. I suppose the nurses could've done the tests and given Dr. Hunter a report, but she wanted to do it herself. She started with my feet and then moved up to my leg, and I could feel all the pokes, but when she started poking my chest and left arm, I couldn't feel the toothpick. This was very surprising. I had full sensation on the right side of my body, but couldn't move either my arm or my leg, but it was the exact opposite on my left side. Both my left arm and leg were able to move easily, and were actually very strong, but I didn't have any tactile sensation on the left side of my upper body or my left arm.

The next thing Dr. Hunter tried was slipping my arm through a blood pressure cuff and pumping it to see if I could feel it getting tighter and tighter as she pumped it. I could feel the cuff getting tighter, but couldn't feel it on my skin. This confirmed that the loss of sensation was just tactile. Uncle Bob (Dr. Adams) came to see me a few times to check if anything had changed with my breathing, but nothing had changed in that department. I was starting to take the occasional breath on my own but not often enough to be taken off the ventilator.

This was when I wanted to give up. I was going to be confined to a wheelchair all day, every day for the rest of my life. I couldn't talk. I couldn't eat or drink. I couldn't even feel the left side of my body. I was always right-handed, but now I couldn't use my right arm, and my right foot needed a brace. I didn't think there was any point in even living anymore. I shared my thoughts with the doctors and nurses, and they all got together and reassured me that there were many other people in the same or even worse positions than mine and they were all living their lives the way they had to. The doctors told me not to focus on what I couldn't do, but on what I still could do. I agreed with them and told myself that I just had to take whatever life threw at me and live with it.

The doctors wanted to keep me in the hospital for another couple of weeks to do more post-surgery tests, but after six or seven weeks of recovering in the SNU, and being tormented with doctors asking how the surgery had affected me, they discharged me and I was transferred to Canuck Place for more respite and a chance to recover. My parents came with my brother and sister a few times to visit with me and keep me company.

I was using the wheelchair all day, but had to have some assistance from the hospital staff to get around. After I'd recuperated for a while, I started manoeuvring the wheelchair on my own. I did this with only my left leg because my right arm was too weak and I couldn't manoeuvre the wheelchair with just one arm. I'd heard that this was bad for my body, because I was pulling all of my body weight with one leg, but that was the easiest way for me to use the wheelchair. If I used just my left arm to propel it, I would just go around in circles and wouldn't get anywhere.

Now that I was using the wheelchair all day, we would have to make some major changes in our lives. With a steeper-than-steep driveway and the main living area located upstairs, our house was not exactly what you'd call wheelchair-friendly. We would definitely have to renovate it or maybe even move. My parents would also have to buy a new car because we didn't have a wheelchair van.

My parents told me that they had started getting in touch with different architects, occupational therapists, designers and contractors and started showing them our house to decide what changes had to be made. One thing they thought of right off the bat was the floor. We had tile downstairs, and that was okay for the wheelchair, but upstairs was all carpet. Our carpeted floors would definitely have to go to avoid the friction against the wheels the carpet would cause. This was the perfect excuse to replace the floors—the carpets were getting old and were starting to gather dust, and with wooden floors we could easily sweep the dust away.

Another big issue was how I would get upstairs. One of the architects suggested building a kitchen downstairs in the laundry room of our house, so we wouldn't have to worry about getting me upstairs, but my mom didn't want to entertain guests in a laundry room. It would also make the house look too small. They also thought of building some kind of elevator in the middle of the house to bring me upstairs, but that meant making a big gap in the house and losing quite a bit of living space.

My parents initially thought of moving to a one-storey home, but that would mean moving too far away and losing the beautiful view we had from our house in North Vancouver. My siblings and I would also have to change schools, and we didn't want to lose our friends. Another reason we were hesitant to move was that if we wanted to move to a house with only one floor, we wouldn't have much of a selection to choose from. Even in a new place, we would have to do some special renovations to our house and make it wheelchair-accessible. So, after little deliberation, we decided to keep our house and do the necessary renovations to it.

30

GF STRONG

JUST AS I WAS getting settled in at Canuck Place, I was moved to another building, literally right across the street from B.C. Children's Hospital, to start intense rehabilitation and to allow time to finish the renovations at our house. GF Strong was a rehabilitation facility where people aged nineteen and older went for rehab. There was another rehabilitation centre that I could have stayed in because it was associated with B.C. Children's Hospital, but that one was more of a teaching centre for younger children with special needs. I needed more physical rehabilitation than what they offered there, so I was admitted to GF Strong, the adult rehabilitation centre. Although GF Strong was geared more towards adults, they did also have special programs for adolescents and young adults, so that was the ideal place for me to stay while I recuperated from my surgery.

They offered many kinds of therapies to patients at GF Strong—everything from physiotherapy to recreational therapy. With over eighty beds and approximately 550 employees GF Strong is British Columbia's largest rehabilitation centre. You can be admitted as an in-patient, and stay overnight, or go as an outpatient just for the day. Health care professionals such as physiotherapists and occupational therapists offer one-on-one, professional treatment for people who have the most severe and complex injuries. The thing was, they didn't have very many private bedrooms at GF Strong. I would have to share a room with a couple of other people. We were separated by curtains instead of walls, so we didn't have much privacy.

Soon after I was admitted to GF Strong we learned that the ward administrator was being pressured to discharge some patients as soon as possible because there were others who needed the space. The social worker who oversaw my care thought of a few alternatives, but they were not very suitable and we didn't think any of them would work for me.

First, she thought of moving me to a foster home and having me driven back and forth as an outpatient so that they could free up space in the ward, but my mom didn't like that idea. I had just come back from a major brain surgery and was left with many physical changes—I needed a lot of rehabilitation from the professional caregivers. Then the social worker thought of keeping me in an RV outside our house so my parents could care for me while the construction workers continued working on the house. This was the most ridiculous idea I had ever heard. Seriously, putting me in a mobile home with a ventilator and nothing to do all day but stare at the walls. The foster home would have been a better idea, but that still wouldn't be the same as staying in the rehab hospital. My parents finally convinced the ward administrator that I would have to stay as an in-patient at GF Strong.

Every weekday morning while I was staying there, I would wake up to the sound of clapping and cheering as I watched *The Price is Right* on TV with some of the other patients who were sharing the same ward as me. We would watch the popular game show every day before all of our therapy sessions began. At eleven a.m., after the show was over, I would go downstairs with my nurse and start my therapies. I stayed in a special area for patients with spinal cord injuries on the second floor and all the services were on the main floor, so I would have to go down the elevator with my nurse and find my way around the hospital to whichever therapist was scheduled to work with me.

My first appointment of the day was an hour-long physiotherapy session with one of the physiotherapists on call. In our first session, she wanted to do an assessment of how I stood and balanced. I couldn't stand back then, so she thought of exercises I could do in bed instead. Eventually she and a rehab assistant would come upstairs to my room and work on what I could do physically at that moment. They would stretch all four of my limbs in different directions for a while and then do some exercises to develop the range of motion in my right arm. They also got me to work on the range of motion in my left arm. I could do this by myself because my left arm wasn't affected by the surgery in the same way my right arm was. I would tell the physiotherapists when they stretched my legs too far, for it would cause a sharp pain.

I had some trouble just sitting at the edge of the bed and balancing, so that was another thing we worked on. The physiotherapist would push me over in bed and I had to resist her push. It took some time for me to get used to this; when I did, they would make it harder for me by raising the bed so that my feet wouldn't have any support from touching the floor. We would do this every morning and, as with everything, I wanted to improve with this as soon as I could, so I would ask my nurses to do these exercises with me when I had any extra time on my hands.

I told the physiotherapist I was very determined to do whatever it took for me to get back to standing and walking again, and that I would work as hard as I could to achieve my goal. I told her what I was already doing before the surgery at home and at school, and she agreed with some of the things Corine had shown me and showed me some other exercises I could do by myself upstairs in my room. One of them was to lie flat on my back in bed and bend both of my legs so the soles of my feet were face down on my bed. I had to straighten one of them at a time by slowly sliding it down the bed, without moving the other leg, then pull it back up. I had to do this ten times, then alternate legs. It was harder to keep my right leg from falling over because it was my weaker leg. I did these exercises every day so that I could move on to the next level of therapy as soon as I could.

The physiotherapist also wanted me to try bouncing around the physiotherapy room on one of those big exercise balls to better my balance. She got a ball from the back of the physio department, and with the help of my nurse, I transferred myself onto it and started by just balancing. The next step was to start bouncing on it. I soon found out that it was easier to take smaller bounces than bigger ones. When I took bigger bounces, I didn't have as much control over myself and the ball. Then, we had an idea. I asked if I could look into a mirror while I bounced. That helped me gain even more control.

I wanted to be as independent as possible while I was staying at GF Strong, so we also worked on me dressing myself and doing basic self-care like brushing my teeth and washing my hands. I used my left hand for most of this because it was a lot stronger than my right hand, and eventually I got to the point where I was doing most of my care by myself, with great difficulty but a lot of determination.

At one point during my six-month stay at GF Strong, the physiotherapists wanted me to walk five metres with one person assisting me. Five metres was the distance the therapists expected of me, but to me it was my absolute minimum. I wanted to walk as far down the hallway as possible, even if I was tripping over my feet.

31

THE NEXT STEPS

WHEN MY PHYSIOTHERAPY appointment was finished, I would go right next door, to the occupational therapy department, to talk with a rehab consultant about getting a wheelchair. The occupational therapist I was working with had already taken measurements of my height and weight to help her decide what size wheelchair I needed for the long run. I was outgrowing the wheelchair they gave me at the hospital, and needed a bigger and sturdier one with all the extra gizmos now that I needed a wheelchair all day.

As we were growing up, my mom always made sure that Ashkan, Maya and I had good manners, so whenever I would meet with any doctors or therapists, I made sure to be as polite and pleasant as I could. I was a happy and cheerful kid, even though I had just lost so many of my abilities, and had pleasant conversations with the therapists who were working with me. This was one reason why everyone at GF Strong loved having me as their client. Another was that I was always open to trying new things.

I tried manoeuvring with the few model wheelchairs they had in the occupational therapy department; I was happy with some of them, but wanted to see what other models were available for me to try. The occupational therapist knew of a company that made different kinds of wheelchairs, so she started ordering in some wheelchairs for me to try. The first one she wanted to try was a power wheelchair, but I couldn't use electric wheelchairs because of my double vision and seizures. Dr. Williams had already warned me that I would most probably always have to use manual wheelchairs. If I had a power wheelchair and I had a seizure, I could go in all directions, possibly running into walls or falling down stairways without any control. We decided to stick with a manual chair, but we all knew it had to be more durable than my last wheelchair.

The first manual chair the occupational therapist ordered was a heavy-duty wheelchair that had a blue frame and reinforced construction to accommodate special needs. It had a strong stainless steel frame that could support up to 450 pounds. As soon as I saw it, I knew it wouldn't be the one for me because I was nowhere near that size and didn't think I would ever grow to be that big. The problem was, it was too wide, and could probably fit two of me side by side in the seat. It was too wide to fit through some of the doorways upstairs, let alone the narrow walkways we had at home. It would probably scratch the walls a lot and that would all be my fault. I asked to try a different one.

The next wheelchair we tried was a special one that had the big wheels at the front. The occupational therapist told me that manoeuvring this one would be a little different because the wheels were backwards; it would be like riding in the opposite direction. I had never heard of this type of wheelchair so I was very excited to try it. My parents were visiting on the day it arrived, so we all went down to the OT department together.

At first glimpse, it looked very strange. The big wheels were popping out at the front of the chair and the small ones were hiding at the back. It didn't have a headrest, and I knew I needed one because of the suctioning, so this model didn't appeal to me very much. The occupational therapist said they could easily install a headrest for me, so I started to consider the chair again. I tried wheeling it around the hospital, but kept getting stuck. This was because I wasn't used to riding with the big wheels at the front. My parents tried to push me around with the chair, but they didn't like how it manoeuvred either. Having the wheels backwards was like riding in reverse, and it wasn't working for me. I didn't think anybody would want this kind of chair because it was so different from all the others. Why was it even on the market?

The next thing the occupational therapist thought of was getting a wheelchair that either reclined or tilted back to relieve some of the pressure off my buttocks and back. The next chair they brought in for me to try was relatively big and comfortable with a backrest that had enough support for me to rest in all day. It tilted back by up to 60 degrees just by squeezing the handrail like you would squeeze the brakes of a bicycle. Another thing I liked about it was that it was very easy to manoeuvre. I tried riding around the hospital with it and found that it turned on a dime. My parents tried pushing me up and down the hallways with it and they also preferred it to the others.

I really liked this wheelchair but there was one problem. The cushion was too hard and was not very comfortable; it felt like I was sitting on a piece of solid wood. The sales representative said that wasn't a problem because she could offer softer materials for me to sit on, and she brought in different sorts of cushions for me to try. After trying a few, I decided the gel cushion was the most comfortable, so all they had to do was measure the cushion and fit it into the seat. It may have taken a lot of trial and error, but I finally found the wheelchair that best suited my needs.

It may have taken a couple of weeks to decide, and a couple more weeks to ship the one I chose, but I had found the perfect wheelchair I could rely on. I may have been a little picky, but at least I picked the wheelchair that worked best for me.

Once I had my "Cadillac of all wheelchairs," as the sales representative called it, I didn't need the other one, so we took it back to B.C. Children's Hospital; I didn't throw it over the bridge like I had wanted to. It was a bit scratched up, but hopefully they could repair it at the hospital and give it to somebody else.

It was very easy to get used to my new wheelchair because it felt so comfortable. It had leather armrests and an adjustable headrest that I could move to whichever height or angle I wanted. The footrests were also adjustable, so I could switch them to different lengths. If I had to criticize one thing, it would be that I couldn't tilt it myself because the control for the tilt feature was at the back of the chair. If I wanted to tilt the chair, I had to ask somebody to tilt it for me.

Ever since the surgery, my right heel was very misaligned, which made it harder for me to stand and balance on my own. We had to find a way to help that, and the only thing the occupational therapist could think of was to make a brace for my right leg to support my foot and keep it in my shoe properly.

They measured my foot and delivered a brace. To put it on, I had to sit at the end of my bed or at the edge of a chair so that a nurse could fit the brace in place. Sometimes it didn't fit properly, especially on the first try, but after a little wiggling around on my foot, and sometimes re-doing the brace completely, the nurses could put it on with ease. The brace really made a difference in the way I stood and how I balanced. It was a major necessity in my new life. My big goal at GF Strong was to stand on my own again, and the brace was the main thing that helped with that.

Another thing I would do at GF Strong was recreational therapy. I would get together with a few of the younger patients and the rec therapist, and we would all go into one of the extra rooms upstairs to either talk and chill out or play games together. We always stayed close to the nurse's station, just in case I had a seizure or if I needed a nurse for anything else.

We sometimes shared stories of why we were staying at GF Strong, and sometimes just played board games all afternoon. The sessions were usually in the evenings, so we would also get a big-screen TV and watch some shows like *The Simpsons* and *Law & Order*. We were all still getting over the cancellation of *Friends*, my favourite TV show ever. There was an NHL lockout that year, so there weren't any hockey games for us to watch. I couldn't think of a worse time to be staying in a hospital for this long.

I felt a little lonely while I was staying at GF Strong, because I was the only teenager in the whole hospital. It looked like almost all the other patients were old enough to be my parents or maybe even my grandparents. There were a few other people in wheelchairs in my recreational therapy group, but they didn't have tracheostomies or ventilators like I did. There was one lady there who had a simple accident at home, but suffered a big disability because of it. She just slipped on the staircase, but hit her neck and therefore suffered from paralysis from the neck down. She also had to have her house renovated, and was waiting for all of that to finish, so some of us were in the same boat.

I told everyone how much I liked to play Scrabble, and that it was very hard to beat me when I was playing competitively; that was why they dubbed me the "Scrabble King" at Canuck

Place. We played countless games of Scrabble, and then some other board games that I wasn't as familiar with. One of the other games we played was a simple two-player game called Mancala. It consisted of forty-eight small glass stones and a small wooden board with twelve cups carved into it. The game starts with four stones in each cup, and players take turns picking up the stones and dropping them, one by one, into the next cup in a counter-clockwise direction.

The recreational therapist recommended this game to me because she thought it would improve my fine-motor skills by requiring me to pick up and control the stones in my hand. I didn't bother trying to use my right hand with this game, because I knew that it would be impossible considering I had absolutely no control or strength in it.

We didn't only play board games during our recreational therapy sessions; we would also go on group outings to one of the many beaches and parks Vancouver is famous for. The rec therapist would get in touch with BCMOS (British Columbia Mobility Opportunities Society) and arrange weekly outings for us. BCMOS is an independent non-profit society dedicated to making it possible for people with significant physical disabilities to access British Columbia's great outdoors through wilderness recreation. They offer many types of activities though BCMOS, programs that range from hour-long hikes to challenging treks up and down outdoor trails, which would not be possible without the strenuous help of their many dedicated volunteers.

GF Strong had many hikes scheduled for us with BCMOS. Many of them required me to use the "Trailrider," a kind of wheelchair that can go off-road and tackle any kind of uneven terrain, and which was supposed to be the backbone of BCMOS programs. Apparently people using Trailriders have reached the peak of Mount Kilimanjaro twice, once in 2002, and again in 2006. It is also versatile and folds down to a very compact size, making it easy to fit it into the back of the big truck we took to our hikes.

We would all drive out of town and into the wilderness and start hiking up and down those dark forest trails. The team of volunteers had different-sized foam pads to use as headrests and body supports and other equipment to ensure comfort. There was always one volunteer pushing the wheelchair at the back and another pulling it from the front. The single-wheel design of the Trailrider made it easy to navigate some of the narrower trails and its lightweight aluminum frame made it easy for the volunteers to manoeuvre.

Although the Trailrider was capable of going off-road, we could also take it to public parks and beaches where the walkways were all paved and there weren't any physical obstacles in our way. On many occasions we spent the day at one of the big and popular parks in Vancouver. We had a few outings at Stanley Park and even more at Kitsilano Beach, even when the weather wasn't as good as I had hoped it would be.

Sometimes we would pack a picnic for those of us who could eat, and take a short break for lunch after hiking in the forests a while. The lunches were simple: sandwiches from the cafeteria at GF Strong, juice boxes or bottles of Coke and maybe some fruits. I had my feeding tube run by gravity, suspended from an IV pole attached to my wheelchair. And sometimes, we ran into other people hiking in the forests or jogging along the sea wall, and we said a quick hello before we headed back to our temporary home.

32
THE RENOVATIONS

MY MOM CAME to visit me five or six times a week while I was recovering from this most recent brain surgery at GF Strong. One day, while I was working on my physiotherapy, she started updating me on the renovations that were going on at home. The designers and construction workers who were taking responsibility for making our house more wheelchair accessible were making more and more progress. They had decided what changes they had to make, but the question was where to start. Should they do the easy things first, or save them for last?

Changing the floors and widening the doorways were the simpler ideas, but the exciting thing was that they had thought of a way to get me upstairs. One of the architects my parents consulted made up his mind that he had to make room for a mechanical lift to bring me up, but he was still deciding where to put it. If he put it in the garage it would go up into the kitchen and take away room in the kitchen, which was already small enough to start with. Then we wouldn't have room for a kitchen table, so my family would have to eat their meals in the formal dining room. The other places in the house where the architect thought of putting the lift would cause other problems.

At last he thought of extending our house and putting the lift in the laundry room. I would enter the lift from the laundry room downstairs and hold a switch to take it upstairs. Somebody would have to open the door of the lift from the outside for me, and then I could enter through the French doors in the living room on the second floor. The builders would just have to extend our porch so there would be enough room for me to manoeuvre. My parents had to get a special permit from City Hall to build this, but once the representatives heard of my situation they approved it right away.

One of the other big projects they had to figure out was the bathroom. We needed a bathroom big enough to accommodate the wheelchair, but which bathroom should they modify? We had one downstairs and two upstairs, one of which was in the master bedroom, so that one was out. But we still had two others to choose from.

My mom told me that since one of the bedrooms downstairs was right beside a bathroom, it would be best if that became my new room. Then the construction workers could connect my room and the bathroom with a private door and I could wheel myself into the bathroom from my bedroom with the wheelchair or a commode. This bedroom was also bigger than the other ones, so there would be more room for my wheelchair and ventilator.

The bathroom would have to be completely redone. This would probably be the most complex part of the renovations. The tub, the sink and the toilet would all have to be removed in order to line and retile the floors and walls to make it all waterproof. At this point it was decided that the sink had to be installed outside the bathroom to make more space for the wheelchair or commode inside, which required quite a bit of additional work.

My mom considered doing more work upstairs too, including removing one of the walls so the walkways wouldn't be as narrow, but then she thought that if they did this, the dining room would look too small and the house would look too open. We would also have to get rid of the piece of artwork that was hanging from the wall and she would prefer not to lose it.

My family was still looking for a wheelchair van for me, but there was not much to choose from: at the time only the Pontiac Montana, Dodge Caravan, Dodge Grand Caravan and Ford Windstar were wheelchair convertible. My parents' first instinct was to get a Grand Caravan because it was the most popular, but we were just starting to look. Honda and Toyota were just coming out with wheelchair-accessible vans, but those ones were very expensive and out of our budget. The conversion alone cost over $25,000.

They'd heard that the manual ramps were easier to control than the automatic ones because the automatic ramps could get jammed easily and would need more maintenance, so my parents were looking for a van that could be controlled manually. Because of our driveway and how steep it was, they wanted a van with a side entry instead of a rear entry, which most wheelchair vans came with. If they got one that opened at the back, and tried to bring me out of the van at the top of the driveway, I would easily roll down the driveway and probably injure myself. My parents hadn't yet decided on a van for me, but they still had a long time until the renovations finished and I was ready to come home. My mom was sure that it would be very hard to drive a van up our steep driveway, so she also thought of redoing parts of it to smooth it out.

My mom had another story to share with me, but it wasn't concerning the renovations. My family had had unexpected visitors the other day. She told me that because the floors were being redone, the builders and renovators had to store a lot of our furniture and other household items in boxes and keep them in the garage. She told me that one day when she came home from visiting me, she noticed that all of my dad's CDs had been torn out of the box he kept them in and were scattered all over the garage and driveway.

She looked inside and noticed paw prints in our dusty garage. The garbage can was toppled over and some of its contents were leaking. My mother quickly recognized the prints as bear paws. When she went inside to inform the workers, they told her that earlier they had seen a mama black bear and three of her cubs rummaging through the garage, looking for food or anything else. They must have smelled the garbage and come looking for it. There was a community rule about keeping all garbage inside for exactly this reason, but the workers had wanted to keep the garage door open so they'd have easier access to their tools.

As soon as the renovators saw the bears once again, they dropped whatever they were doing and slowly backed up inside the house and locked the door. They told my dad that the bears were right in the middle of the garage, and he started to dial Animal Control, but luckily the bears headed back into the forest on their own before the troops got to our house.

We had already had bear warnings and even some sightings in our neighbourhood in the past, but never this close. Maya got a few distant pictures of the bears through the window of our house, but didn't dare get too close to them. It's too bad I wasn't there to see the bears for myself, for I had never seen a live bear before except when I saw two in captivity on Grouse Mountain with everybody from Canuck Place, but I definitely had never seen one out in the open like that.

33

GOING HOME

NOW THAT THE architects and contractors had decided what changes had to be made to our house, it was just a matter of waiting until they finished with everything before I could go back home. I just had to play the waiting game for the next little while. I went on some more hikes with BCMOS, but that wasn't the only thing I did to keep me entertained. I also did things to keep my mind busy. My grade ten science teacher kept sending me all of the homework that I missed in class, and I did some of it just by looking through the textbook and answering the questions. Whenever I did any of my homework, the nurses had to prop me up at a table with pillows and extra supports because I was too weak to sit up on my own.

I read a lot while I was there, just like I would've at home or at school, and one day one of the nurses encouraged me to start reading some of James Patterson's books because she knew that I liked reading mystery and suspense novels. The next time my uncle came to visit me, he picked up a selection of James Patterson's books from the library for me to read. I found that some of them were so good that I couldn't put them down. I liked these books so much that I even read some twice over.

I already had a TV and VCR in my room that my parents had brought from home so that I would have the freedom to watch the shows and movies I wanted on my own time. My uncle had already sent me a bunch of my favourite videos for me to watch before going to sleep, so I had those to keep me entertained for a while. He sent me a lot of *Mr. Bean* videos that I shared with the other people who were staying in the same area of the hospital as me. We watched these and numerous other videos on the small television that my parents had set up for me in front of my bed until late at night.

I knew I had to put up with being in a hospital environment for at least the next few months, but didn't know how much more of it I could take. At least I had already stayed in hospitals for months at a time, so I was used to this kind of setting. I was starting to build relationships with the nurses who were taking care of me, and that helped with my lengthy stay at GF Strong, but it still wasn't the same as being at home.

My family and friends came very often to be with me, especially my grandmother, so the only times I was really alone were in the evening, when I was watching TV, and when I went to sleep at night. There may have been the odd day here and there when everybody was busy at home or work, but I usually had visitors very regularly.

My parents even brought Spunky a couple of times just for fun. One thing about GF Strong was that they permitted small dogs and other small pets into the hospital as long as they were on a leash. One time when they brought him, though, he was in my bed, snuggling with me, and he suddenly jumped off and made his way into one of the elevators across the hall. Luckily, the leash was still attached to Spunky's collar, and the end of it didn't get trapped in the elevator, so one of the nurses just pressed the button that opened the elevator door and pulled him out.

During my last few weeks at GF Strong, I went shopping with my mom to buy thank you presents for some of my therapists and nurses. We bought a necklace for my main physiotherapist and some boxes of chocolates for everyone else. I made a thank you card for the nurses and watched one last movie with everybody who was sharing the ward with me. I knew everybody was enjoying the television set that my parents bought for me, so I left it and some videos when I left the hospital.

My recovery at GF Strong went very well, thanks in part to all of the care and therapy I received from all the staff. Something else that helped was that I wasn't the kind of person who would just give up on something because it was too hard to achieve. I would continue to persevere until I got what I wanted, which was usually going from one point in my therapy to another. That was what really made a difference in my recovery.

My family finally came to pick me up from GF Strong in June 2005, about six months after I had been admitted to the rehabilitation centre. They drove up to the parking lot in our new grey Pontiac Montana with Ashkan and Maya sitting in the back. Just like they promised, my parents got a van with a side entry instead of a rear entry. If I was sitting in the back, I would be more isolated from my family, but with me sitting in the middle I was more part of the group. I said one last goodbye to the hospital staff with whom I'd stayed for so long and I went home to our newly wheelchair-accessible house.

When we got home, my parents started showing me everything that had been modified since I was there last in December of the previous year. First was the small lift in the garage that I would use to get into the house. The designers and contractors decided that a lift would work better than a ramp, which would compromise storage space that was being used for my supplies.

As soon as I went inside, I noticed that not much had changed with the computer room, except that the floors were now hardwood instead of carpet. Then I went into my new bedroom and saw how my parents had rearranged the room to fit a hospital bed, desk, closet, dresser, a small bookshelf and my ventilator all into one bedroom and still saved room for my nurses to have enough space to do everything they needed to do. Another door connected to the bathroom where I could wheel through with my wheelchair or my commode.

In the laundry room I saw the lift I would use to get upstairs. Every time I needed to use it, one of my parents or nurses would open the door for me, and then I could wheel in on my own. I would then have to hold the switch until I got upstairs, and again someone would hold the door for me to roll out. It was the same thing going downstairs, except I had to back in to the lift and hold the switch the opposite way. It was the same kind of contraption we had in the garage, just the doors were different and it was a longer lift.

I used the lift to get upstairs for the first time, but the only major changes I saw to the upstairs of the house were the wooden floors. My parents told me they had widened some of the doorways for my wheelchair and had extended the porch, but I didn't notice that at first glance. They had also repainted some of the walls to a slightly different shade of green, but that didn't register with me either. It had been so long since I had been home last that I couldn't imagine the "before and after" picture in my mind.

34

SAILING AT THE BEACH

IT WAS THEN that Ashkan became more involved in my care. My parents started to "trach-train" him and taught him how to suction me. Now that I was in a wheelchair, I needed more care, so Ashkan and Maya started learning how to help out more with some of the new circumstances our family was faced with. Maya was only nine years old back then, so she was still too young to take on the same responsibilities that Ashkan did. Maya helped out by calling for my parents whenever I needed them for anything.

My brother started suctioning me and helping with some of the physiotherapy exercises I'd brought home from GF Strong. One of the exercises I had to do to improve my balance was to stand on my own and then have Ashkan push gently on my chest and shoulders while I resisted his push and then slowly sat down on my chair by myself. Another was for me to stand up and take a step forward with one leg and hold that position for a few seconds. Ashkan was just about my size, and maybe even a little bigger than me, so standing with him wasn't really a problem once he learned my routine. He also helped with the exercises I did in bed every morning and by pushing my wheelchair around town for me. I always manoeuvred my wheelchair myself when we were home but needed some assistance when we were out on the sidewalks.

This was an interesting development in our relationship, and one that not many siblings are faced with. That may have helped bring us together again. Sometimes it wasn't easy, and I only turned to Ashkan if no one else was available to help me, but looking back now, I realize that it was so important that the whole family took on a share of the work, because there was no way that my parents and I could handle everything on our own.

We had been told that this last brain surgery would have to be my last. The tumour had been de-bulked, but there was still no guarantee that it would stop growing. Dr. Hunter had suggested that we use chemotherapy soon after I recovered from the surgery in an attempt to kill the rest of the tumour or at least stop it from regrowing. The doctors had just been informed that there was a clinical trial for a new kind of chemotherapy for brain tumours, which was produced from periwinkle plants. I was eligible for the trial, so I started another round of chemotherapy treatment as soon as I got home. I was one of the first patients at B.C. Children's Hospital to get this new chemotherapy.

This time we put the chemotherapy into a vial form so that my mom could give it to me through my G-tube. Every night, my mom had to dress up in a gown and wear gloves and goggles to protect herself from the chemo, and then give me the dose before I went to sleep. We didn't want to give this responsibility to the nurses because of the risks involved with chemotherapy.

The chemo may have slowed me down a bit, but at least it was summer and school was over. I only got four months of schooling that year, so I was debating whether I should redo grade ten altogether. My parents told me not to worry about school, but I was more of the studious type of person, so I was a little worried about falling behind. I thought about my studies a little bit more and decided that I could just review the curriculum at home and then move on with my classmates the next year.

I stayed home with Ashkan a lot that summer, partly because of the effects of the chemotherapy treatment and partly because I was reviewing the school curriculum. But I still made time to get outside in the sun and enjoy myself with my family. There was a sailing club for disabled people at one of the beaches in Vancouver, and my mom got me involved with that. The DSABC (Disabled Sailing Association of British Columbia) is a non-profit organization that allows sailors with quadriplegia, paraplegia and other significant physical disabilities to sail independently or with a volunteer. Adapted sailing started in Canada in 1989 and is now one of the fastest-growing sports for people with disabilities. We booked some sails with them and I went out into the water in a sail boat for a couple of hours with one of their volunteers, who was a qualified sailor. I met some members who just came out for a sunny afternoon of leisure activity, and others who were competitive sailors and sailed for prizes.

Another non-profit organization that provided fun and activities for people with disabilities who were looking to get out in the fresh air was Power To Be Adventure Therapy. They go for hikes with small groups of youths and their families who are faced with hardships in their lives. They also had the Trailrider like BCMOS did, as well as another wheelchair that could go off-road called the ORC (off-road chair). It is durable enough to go into the forests and up and down trails, just like the Trailrider does. On the day the ORC was released to the public, the mayor of North Vancouver gave a public speech and told everybody what this newly developed recreational wheelchair meant for hiking even in non-wheelchair-accessible areas. I went to this meeting with my mom and had a chance to interact with others who were going to take part in these activities.

In addition to going on hikes with Power To Be, I got involved with their kayaking program that took place in Deep Cove's beach area. When I went kayaking with them I had to walk down the beach, which was at first very hard for me, and then sit in the front seat of the two-person kayak as one of their volunteers paddled for me from the back seat. I tried to do some of the paddling myself, but I don't think it helped much.

My mom taught the volunteers what to do if worse came to worst and I had a seizure while out on the water, but the chances of that happening were slim and she reassured them that it probably wouldn't happen. I would go out on the water for a couple of hours with a small group of others taking part in this experience and then head back to the beach where we would just chat for a while before going back home. Power To Be also has a program for the participants to go camping and learn all about nature and outdoor-life skills, but I couldn't take part in these overnight events because of my tracheostomy and my need to use a ventilator at night.

I am very grateful for all of the good times the DSABC and Power To Be have provided. It's good to know that they are there for so many people.

35

BACK TO SCHOOL

THERE WERE SOME drastic changes in my schooling when I returned to school in September. Things were different physically, psychologically, emotionally and cognitively. It's true, I did have the tumour in my brain when I started high school, but it wasn't slowing me down when I was in grade eight. I was always a high achiever, trying to get the best grades out of the whole class, but that was when the tumour was under control. At that point, I wasn't under the effect of so many medications, I wasn't recovering from an aggressive surgery, and, most importantly, I didn't have to deal with being on chemotherapy.

Now a lot of things were different. My memory wasn't the same and neither was my attention span. I was continuing to attend my classes with Laura, and she was continuing to take notes for me as my scribe; I still had Mr. Inkster as my main LSC teacher; and, best of all, Allyson was still making time to help stand with me in the gym. When I'd first told them that I would be away for some time due to this big surgery, they were all worried sick about me. They didn't think they would ever see me again. But now that I was back at school, a big wave of relief came over them.

I was back at school now, but I wasn't paying as much attention in class as I used to, and I was just letting Laura do most of my homework for me. I really had to strive hard to get the same grades as before, but this was too much for me, so in a way, I stopped caring so much about school.

Then one day Mr. Inkster called my mom and me in to have an important meeting with him. Laura and some of the other LSC teachers I worked with attended the meeting too. He brought up the fact that I was starting to become a different type of learner. I agreed with him and confessed that I wasn't putting as much effort into my schooling as I used to. My education was no longer my number one priority; it had gone considerably far down the scale. I'd just come back from one of the most dangerous operations imaginable, and I was going through all these crucial changes in my life, so I felt like a completely different person. Before the surgery, I was more motivated by marks, but since I'd come back to school, I was becoming more of a self-motivated student. I was going to my classes more for the sake of learning, and not just trying to beat everyone else with the highest grades. At first I was in deep denial about my situation, but as soon as I accepted that I wasn't the same person as I used to be, I was able to continue with my schooling more comfortably.

When Allyson and I got together, I told her what the physiotherapists from GF Strong were expecting me to do, so we started trying to do those exercises. I was definitely weaker than before the surgery, so my standing wasn't the same as it was the last time we had worked together. I sometimes cheated, and didn't do everything I was told to because I occasionally felt like I had to take a break from exercising. Everybody at GF Strong knew how determined I was, but they didn't want me to strain myself too much, so it was actually better for me to take breaks from exercising every now and then.

I had a new nurse with me after I was discharged from GF Strong. Nichole was her name, and she at least had some previous experience with tracheostomies and ventilators, so it was easier for her to take care of me compared to the other nurses who were just getting started with trachs and vents. Nichole really knew what she was doing with the tracheostomy, so it just took a couple of days of orientating her to my routine and she worked very well with me by herself.

My care was complex for Nichole, especially the tracheostomy changes, but the fact that I was older and I could direct my care made everything easier for her. It also helped that I was on the ventilator only part-time, so she didn't have to be as wary with me as with her other clients who were younger and needed a ventilator all day. I made a point of wearing my speaking valve more often so that she could understand me more easily.

Like all of my previous nurses, Nichole was always worried about my seizures, worried about when they would occur and if she would have time to bag me with the Ambu bag, but I didn't have too many seizures with her during the day, so things weren't as bad as she had expected them to be.

Unfortunately, the chemotherapy was still getting to me. Some days I felt too weak and tired to stand, so we skipped the standing exercises I did at school during my spare block and Nichole took me outside to get some sun and fresh air. We would walk around the block for about a half hour and then head back to the school before the beginning of my next class. This was usually part of my daily routine with Nichole.

After school I still had a little bit of time with Nichole at home before her shift finished, so we would play games until she had to leave. I used to play a lot of chess whenever I came home from school, and I wanted to play with Nichole, but she had no idea how to play the game. I had a beginner's set at home that showed you how each piece moved, and I tried using that to show her my strategy of winning, but she didn't catch on very fast. Nichole's nursing care was better than her chess skills, and that was a higher priority for me.

Even though I had Laura working with me all day at school, Mr. Inkster wanted to make things easier for me, so he got SET-BC (Special Education Technology British Columbia) to send one of their representatives to assess my needs and possibly make it easier for me to do my schoolwork independently. When the representative came, he and the school therapists asked me what they could provide to help me do my work more independently. I told them that a laptop might help because I couldn't write anymore. I thought this would probably make it easier for me to take notes in class without depending on Laura.

The thing was, I couldn't type very fast, and I would have to press just one key at a time when I typed, so maybe even a laptop wouldn't do the trick. They thought they had a solution for that: special software to recognize my voice so that I could just talk out loud and the computer could type whatever I said in for me. But there was another problem with that idea: because of the trach, my voice was too soft for the computer to recognize it clearly enough. It was a little better when I wore the speaking valve, but it still didn't recognize everything I said.

Then Mr. Inkster and the SET-BC representative had the idea of getting a different type of software to download onto my new laptop. This one was meant to predict the next word I wanted to type. I just had to type in the first few letters of a word, and the computer would give me a bunch of options to choose from. Now most smartphones have predictive keyboard technology, but it was a new thing when I was in grade eleven and the perfect tool for me to use at school and when I did my assignments at home. Although this technology helped me with typing on the computer, I still had all the other aspects of school to deal with.

We had decided that I was going to stop taking classes in French that year, but was going to attend the same school to be with the same classmates I had been with since grade eight. I hadn't spoken any French for almost a year and was starting to forget my third language. I was going to stop French immersion in grade twelve anyway, so why not just stop now? Plus, the new software I had on my laptop only recognized the English language.

When I was choosing my classes for that year I noticed that one of the teachers was teaching a law class, so I signed up for that. I had no intention of going into the legal field after high school, but I thought this class would be more interesting than biology or chemistry or any of the other sciences. I already knew a thing or two about law courtesy of *Law & Order*, so I felt confident that I would do all right in this class.

There was also an art class available, and Mr. Inkster and Nichole recommended that I try that. I didn't think I would want to because I knew I would have to do everything with one hand only. Then I remembered that art therapy was one of the recreational activities we did at GF Strong, and I had seen how some of the patients who had complete quadriplegia painted just by holding a paintbrush in their mouths and moving their heads from side to side, so I thought that I could at least try painting with my left hand even if I didn't use it to write. This was one example of being inspired by people in worse positions than me who still did not give up. I had a great art teacher who showed us different drawing and painting techniques to express ourselves artistically. I tried to draw self portraits and even some landscapes. I got this idea from admiring the views of the North Shore mountains and the beaches around town from various lookouts around Vancouver. I also remembered all of the paintings we saw in Rome. They were all beautifully painted by the most skilled artists from around the world. I tried to do my own paintings that resembled some of these, but they weren't nearly as good. We were doing fine arts for most of the class, so I didn't need to use my laptop that often.

36
SEPSIS

LATER THAT FALL, after not seeing any of the doctors from B.C. Children's Hospital for over a year, we had another appointment with Dr. Williams, who wanted to see how I was doing since he last operated on me. I told him about how I worked at GF Strong and how we had renovated the house for my wheelchair. All of my side effects from the surgery were still the same as when he assessed me in the hospital. He was expecting me to be weaker than before the surgery because it was such an intense operation, so nothing really surprised him. I may have been a little sluggish on the day of our appointment, but he knew that I was still on the chemotherapy and I'm sure he took that into consideration.

After seeing Dr. Williams for the last time, we moved on to see Dr. Hunter, the neuro-oncologist who put me on the new chemotherapy treatment. She ordered an MRI for that same day to see how it was working, and it showed that the tumour had shrunk to be very narrow and only five centimetres long. So there actually was some good that came out of being on this third round of chemotherapy after all. Dr. Hunter didn't want to risk killing any more of the good cells in my brain with more chemo, so she took me off it after that appointment.

I wasn't going to have another brain surgery to physically de-bulk the tumour, so Dr. Hunter took over for Dr. Williams as my primary doctor. She was mainly just going to keep an eye on the tumour for me and make sure it was under control. I didn't think there was much more she could do, for the doctors had already done all of the available treatments to get rid of the tumour.

Since it was flu season, we were all taking extra precautions not to get sick. We were washing our hands more often and making sure not to contaminate each other. My parents increased my vitamin intake and gave me organic food through my G-tube with hopes of boosting my immune system. My mom started replacing my normal feed with this new vegan and organic diet she had heard about. Unfortunately for me, though, the special diet that was supposed to cleanse my system worked the opposite way.

One day during Christmas break, when I was home watching TV, I had a very intense seizure in the family room and fell off my wheelchair. I toppled over onto my side and an enormous amount of mucus and secretions were pouring out of my mouth and tracheostomy like lava erupting from a volcano. My father heard me pounding on the floor, trying to call for help, and he ran upstairs and saw the position I was in. He immediately called 911, and they sent an ambulance and a fire truck to take me to the hospital. When the firefighters came, they quickly carried me on a stretcher down the stairs, put me into the back of the ambulance and rushed me to Children's Hospital with their lights and sirens blaring at full blast.

When we got to the Emergency ward of the hospital, we quickly checked in and found our way to the ICU. Lucky for me, Dr. Adams was in charge of the ICU that day, and as soon as he recognized me he dropped everything and attended to me without any hesitation. He took my temperature and it turned out that I had a very high fever. He also took my heart rate and noticed that my heart was beating way faster than it should. I was breathing very rapidly, so he put me on a ventilator and adjusted the settings to what I had at home every night. He wanted it to take control of my breathing to calm me down so I wouldn't hyperventilate. If it weren't for him being there, we would've had to call for another respirologist, and who knows what would've happened by the time the other doctor got to me and went through my charts to learn my ventilator settings.

Dr. Adams tried talking to me, and making sure I was alert, but I wasn't responding normally. I was trapped inside some kind of scary seizure and was screaming a lot of crazy nonsense that I wasn't aware of. I was unconscious on and off for the next hour or so, but as soon as I came back to consciousness the ICU nurses took a blood sample from me and found that there was an infection in my blood; this was definitely not a good sign. This meant that I had sepsis, or blood poisoning, a potentially life-threatening condition in which the body fights a severe infection that spreads throughout the bloodstream.

Sepsis usually occurs when the immune system is not working properly due to an illness or because of medical treatments like chemotherapy or steroids. This must have happened because of the chemotherapy I was on earlier and may have also had something to do with bacteria from the organic diet my mom put me on at home. You always have to consider the pros and cons of every kind of medical treatment. The special diet is probably what weakened my immune system, and then the chemo must have taken advantage of it.

Judy was my nurse that day—the same Judy who had known me for many years, since I had first started having nurses at home. She really freaked out when I had that massive seizure and toppled onto the floor. She really thought that that was it for me, but no, I wouldn't go that easy.

Once the doctors and nurses confirmed that I was septic, they re-admitted me to B.C. Children's Hospital for the umpteenth time. This facility and GF Strong were really becoming like second homes to me. I stayed in an isolation room again because the nurses couldn't afford to risk any of my germs spreading and getting to the other patients. Neither did they want to risk getting me sick in any other ways, so they tried to keep me separate from everybody else.

The nurses treated the blood poisoning with loads of antibiotics every morning. I was sure they knew what they were doing by giving me the right medications, but I was beginning to feel suspicious about all the drugs that were considered medicine. All of the other medicines and treatments I got seemed to have their own side effects, so these probably did too. Just look at what the chemotherapy did to me. I wanted to go over to Dr. Hunter's office and tell her about the sepsis, but it may not have been necessary. She may have already heard the news from Dr. Adams, and it probably wouldn't have surprised her. She already knew how dangerous chemotherapy was and what maladies it could cause.

The next few days were nothing new. I received antibiotics through daily IVs, and my blood was slowly getting back to normal. The nurses always pulled off so much hair when they took off the tape for the IVs it was a free personal wax job (not that I wanted one).

The days were long and boring, but that's how it is when you stay in the hospital. There was a TV in the Special Needs Unit that all of the patients shared, but I had to stay in my isolation room at all times. I didn't enjoy daytime TV anyway, except maybe for game shows. I compensated by listening to the CDs my parents brought me from home. My favourites were Eric Clapton, Bob Marley, Billy Joel, Queen, The Guess Who and The Police. One album didn't get much play, though; I wasn't really a big fan of The Beatles, even though they were probably the most famous band of all time.

I had nothing to do all day but listen to music and read lots of books. This is when I really started to get into James Patterson's books. I even watched the movie *Kiss the Girls,* based on one of Patterson's bestselling Alex Cross books. I had a few family visits while I recovered, but not too many because even they were encouraged not to come into my isolation room.

Approximately ten days after the doctors had found the sepsis, I was cleared to go back home with my bloodstream free of infection. My mom took me off the special diet of all-vegan and organic foods, so my immune system went back to normal. My last admission to Children's Hospital had been shorter than all the other ones, but equally as lonesome.

37

GETTING BETTER

BY SUMMERTIME, I had gained a lot of stability in the core of my body and in both legs, so I started doing more physiotherapy at GF Strong and with Corine every week. I was admitted as an outpatient to GF Strong and worked with Cathy, the outpatient physiotherapist for an hour per visit to the rehab centre. I showed her the exercises I was practising at home, and set a goal to slowly improve my physical state. I wanted to start walking either independently or at least with a walker as soon as possible. I knew it would take a lot to get to that point, but I was ready to do anything and everything I could to achieve my goal. I was sure that working consistently with Cathy and Corine was going to bring me closer to walking again. My high school graduation was coming up the next year, and I sure as hell didn't want somebody pushing me across the stage in a wheelchair. I wanted to walk across like everyone else.

Cathy got me to stand up and took her time to thoroughly assess me, but then thought it was too early for me to even think about walking. I still wasn't steady enough on my feet to stand on my own, let alone to walk, so she gave me some other exercises to do to improve my balance. I had to put one leg in front of the other and try to balance like that for as long as I could without feeling off-balance. I wanted to at least try walking while assisted by the walker, but when I did, I felt very sloppy on my feet. I told her I would do the new exercises at home with my brother and at school with my nurses whenever I got a chance.

The upside to coming back to GF Strong was their focus on making their clients more independent. Cathy showed me a way of transferring myself from my wheelchair to another seat in the house or onto my bed without any assistance. She told me to angle my wheelchair close to the seat I wanted to transfer to and hold my left armrest with my left hand. Then I had to push on the armrest and stand up only half way, like I was crouching down, and quickly pivot across and sit down on the couch or whatever I was transferring onto. The first few tries resulted in me falling to the floor, but with practice I eventually started transferring perfectly on my own. This wasn't exactly what I had come to GF Strong for, but at least it was something I could practise other than just sitting and standing.

When I told Corine about my goal of walking and about my experience with a walker at GF Strong, she thought of a new way to get me more active. She came up with a way for me to walk with two people supporting me, one on each side. I always had to take my first step with my stronger leg, which was my left leg, and then try to pick up my right leg and put it ahead of my left leg. She told me not to play catch up with my legs, but to always put one leg ahead of the other and go one step further. We tried to schedule Corine's visits for the days and times the nurses were with me so she could teach them the physiotherapy too.

I had one person holding each of my hands, and whenever I took a step with my left leg, I had to push down on the hand that was supporting my left side. I then had to make sure I picked up my right leg and took it one step ahead of the other one. It was easier to gain control of my right leg by putting the extra pressure on my left hand.

We didn't have very much room in the house to practise inside, but we did what we could and tried walking outside in our cul-de-sac. My grandmother had more room to walk in her house, so every time we went to her house for family get-togethers, I would practise my walking. I wasn't very stable and was only able to take two or three steps before feeling like starting over, but with practice, I started getting better.

Corine knew how badly I wanted to excel, so she even showed me how to go up and down stairs with some help. Again, I had two people supporting me, and when I wanted to take a step up, I had to put my left leg on the stair and push up because it was better for me to put all of my weight on my stronger leg. I tried using my right leg for this, but that definitely wouldn't work; I couldn't handle all of my weight on such a weak leg. It was the same taking steps down; I always had to step with my stronger leg first.

The stairway in our house was too narrow for three people to stand side by side on it, so we had to practise doing the stairs in the quiet community centre close to our house and on the stairs leading up to my grandmother's house. My dad would help me on one side, and my uncle would hold me on the other.

Now that the sun was out and the weather was good again, I had more opportunities to go outside and walk. I wanted to practise as much as possible. I needed two people to walk with me, so Ashkan sometimes volunteered to help me walk outside with Judy or Nichole. He would take my left arm, and the nurse would help me on the right, so that I could push down on his hand. We would walk up and down the cul-de-sac a few times, just like Corine suggested, and then go back home to rest on the couch. Later that summer, Judy went into management at work, so Nichole became my primary nurse. She came more often, so I had more chances to walk and improve in that department.

We scheduled more sailing adventures at Jericho Beach with the DSABC and more kayaking trips in Deep Cove with Power To Be. My family and I also went on more hikes with the Trailrider and the ORC. However, I spent most of my summer working on my physiotherapy, preparing for my high school graduation the next year.

38

GRADUATION

I STARTED SCHOOL IN September just like I would have started any other year, except this was grade twelve and I would be graduating from high school at the end of the year. When my family and caregivers realized what year it was, everyone got all emotional. Nobody thought I would get this far in life, especially with the tumour still not under control, but I wouldn't let that get in the way of getting my high school diploma.

I was very excited about starting to walk again, even though I needed two people assisting me. I taught Allyson the method Corine used to get me more mobile, and she and my nurse started walking with me up and down quiet hallways when we had the chance to work on my physiotherapy during the school day. My main goal was to walk across the stage at the graduation ceremony. I knew I would have to work hard to achieve this goal, but I was prepared to do whatever it took.

When we started to walk, Allyson was baffled by how much walking I could do without falling over or needing to stop and catch my breath. She asked me what was going on and all I said was that I had stopped the chemo. That treatment was the one that affected me the most.

That year everyone at school was starting to understand me better when I spoke without having to use the speaking valve. Before, whenever I went to school, I would put my speaking valve on especially to talk, but now everyone could understand me when I was just wearing the HME. Sometimes it was frustrating when I couldn't be understood without the speaking valve, but that's how it was with everyone, so I couldn't really blame anyone. Everyone needed their time to get used to my tracheostomy and the little voice that I still had.

Early in the month, when the weather was still nice outside, and it was possible to get outside without getting wet, the staff got all of the future graduates of the class of 2007 to go out onto the school's gravel field and assemble in the form of a zero and a seven. They were going to take an aerial view photo of us for the yearbook. I took my place beside some of my classmates at the front of the zero and the photographer took all of the photos from a helicopter that was hovering in the sky above us. This was the first of many graduation events to take place that year.

When we walked at school, the nurse would hold the back of my jeans, just to stabilize my hips, and would also hold my hand and help me walk down the hallway with Allyson. I was also walking at home and at my grandmother's house with my dad and Ashkan, so I was slowly getting better with that. Practice always made perfect with me.

We had to take our graduation photos early in the year. There was a cameraman who came to the school to take our pictures. We didn't have to dress up or anything, for we were wearing the graduation gowns over our everyday clothes. We did have to write a little quotation to go with our photos, which the staff were going to read aloud on the loudspeaker as each graduate crossed the stage at our graduation ceremony. Everybody wrote about how much they enjoyed school at Argyle and about the friends they made. Mine was similar to everyone else's, but I also thanked everyone who helped me make it to this point in my life. Some students attached a baby photo of themselves to go in the yearbook, but that was optional, so I didn't do it.

There was a grad survey around the end of the year, in which we chose the most random categories you could think of, and voted for the graduate who best suited that category. There was everything from who was the loudest party animal to who had the best eyes to who had the best tan. I was voted the nicest grad, and everyone elected Allyson as the grad most likely to fall asleep in class, which was hard to believe considering the grades she got in school.

At the beginning of the year, Mr. Inkster told everyone that the school was going to rent out a theatre downtown for the graduation ceremony. When that day came, my dad drove our whole family to the theatre for my big day. My parents and siblings had their seats on the right side of the stage, and all of the graduates were seated in the first few rows of the audience. It was very humid in the theatre, just like I was expecting it to be, but I wasn't too hot. Mr. Inkster had already warned me that it would be very warm in the theatre, with all the guests in the same auditorium, so it would probably be best for me not to wear my suit jacket if I was planning to wear a suit. I definitely didn't want to have a seizure at the ceremony, so I chose to just wear a dress shirt and my graduation gown over it.

The theatre was very big and was perfect for our graduating class, which was the biggest Argyle had ever seen with over 360 graduates. The only problem for me was going to be that the stairs leading up to the stage were very narrow. Since I wanted to walk across the stage, I would have one person helping me on each side but the stairs were too narrow to accommodate three people at once. We had already planned that since the stairs were so narrow, and because the graduates were being announced alphabetically and I was going to be one of the first called, I would enter the theatre through the back entrance and sit backstage with Ashkan and wait until my name was called.

There were only ten or eleven students ahead of me, so the wait wasn't too long. When it was my turn to cross the stage, I stood up with Ashkan and started to walk. As soon as I was on my feet and walking, everyone who was graduating with me jumped up in a standing ovation. As soon as they stood up, the remaining two thousand people in the audience did too. I was too focussed on walking without tripping over my feet to completely notice this, but I could hear the cheering and applause very clearly. I crossed the stage, shook hands with the principal, and then took another graduation picture just for good measure.

Our graduation banquet was held immediately after the ceremony. I sat with my parents while they ate their dinner. Allyson and her parents were sitting at another table, not too far from us. I went over to her table to introduce myself for the first time, and tell her parents how Allyson was the best friend I had made at Argyle. I told them how much she helped me during high school and how much I appreciated her help. They said that I was a real inspiration to everyone, especially Allyson, and that she was happy to help. After dinner, we all got on the dance floor and danced and socialized until late at night. When it was time to leave, I wished my former classmates well with big hopes for the future.

Finally, after twelve years of school, and many times of feeling unsure if I would live to see another day, I was graduating from high school, ready to start a new chapter in my life.

39

DEAN MACHINE

SHORTLY AFTER MY graduation, my nurse Nichole had to leave us, so we had to find a new primary nurse for me to work with at home. We found a young man, with whom I quickly built a strong relationship. His name was Dean and he was a small guy, who, at a mere five foot five, was pretty short compared to my six feet. I had had male nurses at the hospital and at GF Strong before, but Dean was my first male nurse at home.

Now that I was staying home most days I had a lot of free time on my hands. It helped to have Dean with me because he could think of things for us to do together when I wasn't too busy. This was just one good thing about having him around. Another was that he was younger than any of the other nurses I'd had before, and I preferred having younger nurses because I could relate to them more. Most of my previous nurses were quite a bit older than me, and sometimes I felt like I had one of my parents with me all day long. But that wasn't the case with Dean. It was nice to have someone closer to my age to hang out with and go places with. He had a nice personality that everybody liked, and seemed like the perfect nurse for me.

A few weeks prior to leaving, Nichole orientated Dean, and during his orientation, Dean seemed very confident to be with me by himself. He learned everything very quickly, which displayed his ability to have fun while at work. The only downside was that Dean didn't have a lot of experience with tracheostomies, so I had to guide him through most of my care. Dean had some trouble suctioning me at first, a skill that takes some time to master, even though we do it quite regularly. He also had some problems reading my lips and communicating with me. I sometimes had to repeat myself a few times and even had to use hand signals so he would understand me, but he eventually got the hang of things and started communicating with me more easily.

Despite his size, Dean was very strong, so he could easily take me out of the house on public transit. He was really into protein shakes and keeping fit, so he encouraged me to start working out like he did. We started going to a local community centre, which was just a short walk from my house, and made an appointment with the personal trainer at the gym. She showed us around and taught me which machines I could use with Dean's help. One machine in particular seemed like a good workout for my whole body. It had a reversible seat that I could sit in, then I could strap my feet and hands onto the footrests and handrails, and push the rails back and forth. This machine was very easy for me to use, and it was apparently the only one they had on the North Shore. When I took Corine to the gym and showed her the machine she really liked it and said she would strongly recommend it to any of her other clients.

Soon after I started going to the gym in the community centre, Dean and I found another rec centre in North Vancouver that was bigger and more wheelchair accessible than the one we were used to. This one was a little further away, but it had some different machines I could use and a weight room. It also had a swimming pool in it that could accommodate wheelchairs, so I could also go in the water after my workout. I just had to make sure that I didn't get any water in my trach. Dean and I started going to that one too.

The first little while Dean was like any of my other nurses, but as time went on we became close friends. We would call each other names, make fun of each other, tease each other and even slap high fives. We made up nicknames for each other. My favourite nickname for him was Dean Machine just because it rhymed, and he used to call me Bionic Man or B-Train. I used to call him a "little boy" for fun, and he would respond by calling me a "teenage boy." Our birthdays were only a couple of days apart, so we would also buy each other birthday presents. We had similar senses of humour, so I had a lot of fun with Dean.

40

THE LAST GOODBYES

I SPENT A LOT of free time with Dean by my side. Then, early in the summertime, I had twenty-four-hour nursing coverage at home. I had the whole house to myself for over a week and this was my chance to do whatever I wanted. I had three day nurses working with me on separate days of the week, but Dean came to be with me the most often. We went to see some movies with all of the free time on our hands, but spent most of our time outdoors, either downtown or at the beach. We didn't have to worry about getting home on time because Dean was scheduled to be with me all day anyway, until the night nurse took over late at night.

The Canucks made it far in the playoffs that year, so I went with Dean to a couple of pubs downtown to watch the semifinal games with some of the Canucks' other die-hard fans. Unfortunately, though, our home team lost the best-of-seven series to their playoff nemesis, the Chicago Blackhawks, in game six of the Western Conference semifinals, and with that they were ejected from the playoffs for that year.

I was later re-admitted to GF Strong as an outpatient again to better my physical condition and hopefully start walking comfortably again. I was already sitting, standing and doing other exercises on my feet with ease, so my next goal was to start walking. My appointments were in the early afternoons, so Dean and I had enough time to take the bus to rehab and didn't need anyone to drive us.

I showed Kristy, the outpatient physiotherapist I was working with, what I could do physically, and told her what goals I wanted to achieve. Then she got a walker that she could adjust to my size from the back of the physiotherapy department so I could try it. She told me what position to stand in and how exactly to hold the walker, and we started walking in the hallway. When I first tried the walker, my posture needed a lot of improvement because I wasn't used to walking on my own, but with Kristy's patience and help, and a lot of practice on my part, I quickly improved. I am no longer slouched over when I walk; I can walk easily with the walker standing up straight.

Later in the year, we finally made my last appointments with my doctors, just to finalize everything. Since I was no longer a pediatric patient, my treatment at B.C. Children's Hospital was wrapping up and any appointments would from now on be at Vancouver General Hospital. I went to see Dr. Adams first, and when I went into his office, he did another assessment on me. He asked how I was doing with my tracheostomy, and I told him everything felt the same as usual. I also told him again how much I loved having him as a doctor. I had built a very strong relationship with Dr. Adams since we first met about ten years prior to that appointment. I had him to thank for customizing my cuffed tracheostomy, and he was the one who saved my life when the doctors detected that I was septic. Saying goodbye to Dr. Adams for the last time was like leaving a best friend; it was very hard for me.

My next appointment was with Dr. Hunter, the doctor who oversaw the care for my tumour and seizures. When I met with her she asked about my seizures, which were minimal by then, and then she asked my mom if she wanted her to refer me to an oncologist in the adult world or to another neuro-oncologist. We preferred a neuro-oncologist because we still weren't sure how the tumour would behave in the future, and wanted expert advice for the long run. Dr. Hunter had put me on three different rounds of chemotherapy over the ten-year span that I had been her patient. The first two didn't really do anything to help with my situation, but the third one shrank the tumour by 20 percent. She studied very hard to understand my extremely rare case. It was an honour to have her as my doctor.

I'd already had my last appointments with Dr. Williams and Dr. Robinson a long time before, so we didn't need to see them again. The only thing I saw Dr. Robinson for was my neck, and that problem had been solved about a decade previously, so we had already seen him for the last time long ago. Dr. Williams had done a few surgeries on me since I'd become his patient, and he had helped a lot while consulting about what to do with the tumour. He definitely was one of the best doctors we could find for my condition. When he had first diagnosed me, everyone was scared to death, but the end result wasn't as bad as we had thought it to be.

Our final thing to do before we left the hospital was go over to the ICU and SNU to say goodbye to the nurses who had taken care of me while I was there. We took them boxes of chocolates and thank you cards as tokens of our appreciation. Just before we left, we had our last chat with the main ICU nurses who had trach-trained my parents, and I gave them the gifts we had brought for them, and with that we took our last few steps out of B.C. Children's Hospital.

POSTSCRIPT

ONCE I WAS finished at B.C. Children's Hospital, I started having my appointments at Vancouver General Hospital. Dr. Williams and Dr. Hunter referred me to Dr. Thompson, a neuro-oncologist in consult who worked at VGH and at the B.C. Cancer Agency, and Dr. Adams referred me to Dr. Ride, another respirologist, just at VGH. I was one of the first kids in British Columbia with a tracheostomy to go from childhood to adulthood. I still have to go back to one of the hospitals once or twice a year to get regular MRIs, just to make sure the tumour is stable. There haven't been any concerns with it since my last surgery in 2004.

Nobody knows for sure where the tumour came from or how it started, but some of my doctors think I was born with it. My family could notice all along that something wasn't right with me ever since I was born but we never found anything concrete until I was diagnosed with my tumour in 1998.

A lot of people have asked me how I do it. My best piece of advice is to always stay positive and forget about the negative parts of life. Focus on the good parts in life and try to be happy with what you have. This will keep you happy. One of the most important assets in life is happiness, so try to keep that as a priority. That was what helped me the most, and I am sure that many other people will benefit from it too.

Another key benefit that helped me through my childhood agony was the great amount of patience I had for everything. From lying in MRI machines for hours at a time to lying in hospital beds for days, I needed a lot of patience to endure. Every time I had a doctor's appointment, I knew I would have to sit in the waiting room for a long time until they were ready to see me. After a while it became routine. Patience is, after all, a virtue, and a valuable one at that—it's something we all need in order to succeed throughout life.

Patience was one virtue that helped me get through this whole ordeal, but two other, more essential ones that boosted me forward were faith and love. We have family and friends all over the world, and they were all concerned about me as I grew older, so I had a lot of moral support. Whenever I was going through one of my operations or starting one of my chemotherapy or radiation treatments, they organized twenty-four-hour chain-prayers around the world to pray for me. I thank everyone for all of the love and support I have received throughout my life.

I had to sacrifice a lot because of everything that went on in my life, but one thing I didn't give up was my ability to not let things get to me. Every time I lost one of my natural abilities, I focussed instead on what I could still do, and I just had to accept that I could no longer do the same things as before. When I had to get the tracheostomy, I had no choice but to stop eating and drinking, but after my last surgery, when I needed a wheelchair all day, I had the choice of hanging my head low or trying to regain my strength both physically and psychologically. I chose to challenge myself and regain my strength because I knew it would get me farther in life. I worked hard and did the best I could with everything, and all of that perseverance certainly paid off. I am now twenty-five years old and continuing my education while doing some volunteering in my community and making the most of my surroundings.

Yes, there were some barriers that got in my way as I grew into adulthood, but I didn't let them stop me. I strived hard to get to where I am today. I didn't give up or feel sorry for myself and I certainly didn't limit myself. I always exceeded expectations and never settled for the minimum. If I had, I might not have been able to do the things I can do these days. My neck would be frozen in one place, I would be sitting in a wheelchair all day, unable to stand or walk independently, and I wouldn't be involved with the community in the same way I am today.

Of course, I may not have continued my life in the same way I did if it weren't for all the help and support my family and I have received from everybody in our community. My family has played a big role in my success growing up and reaching my goals, but I would also like to thank my friends, neighbours, therapists, doctors, nurses and everybody else who supported me in many ways over my lifetime.

For some time now, I have been thinking of writing the story about my life, and now that I've written this, I have achieved that goal too.

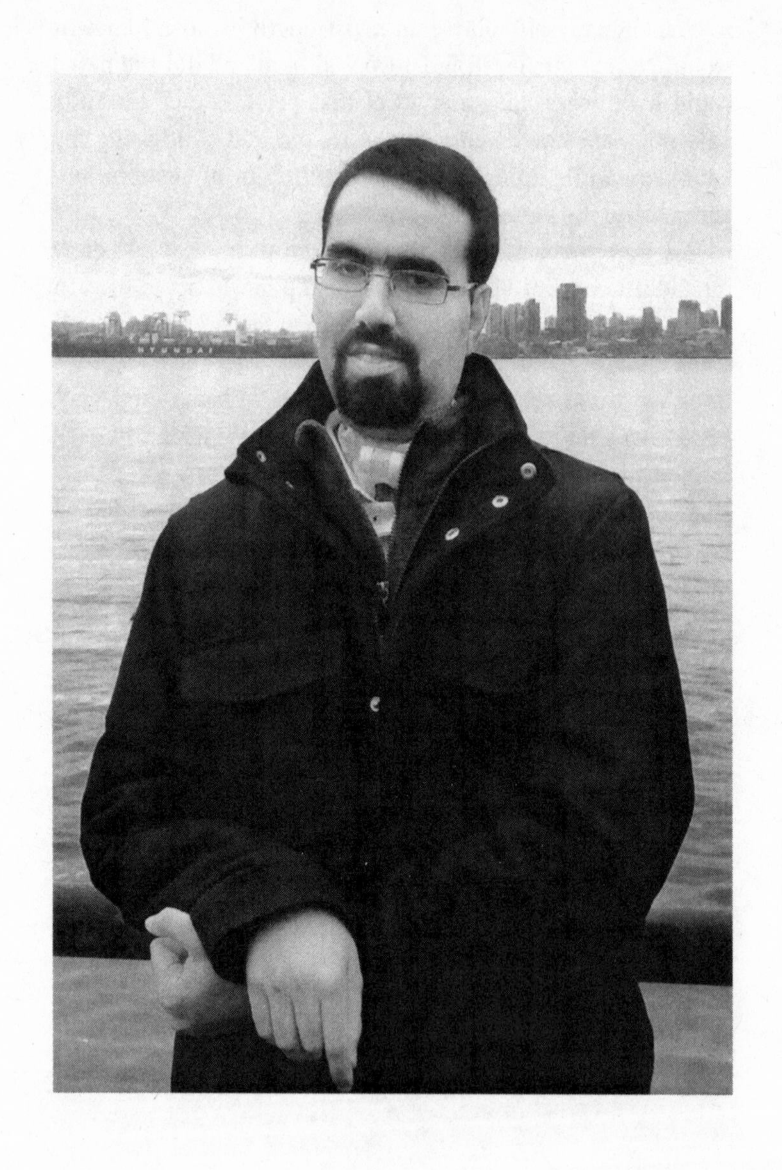

ABOUT THE AUTHOR

BAYAN AZIZI is the first-time author of *Me, Myself and My Brain Stem Tumour.* An avid reader and writer, Bayan started to write a journal of his life story while attending classes at Capilano University and quickly realized his story of surviving a rare brain tumour was a book-length project. Over a period of three years he worked continuously until he had a finished manuscript. The son of Baha'i parents who came to Canada after living in Iran, the UK and Africa, Bayan grew up with his brother and sister in the Mount Seymour area of North Vancouver. He graduated from Argyle Secondary School and attended Capilano University. He is extremely self-motivated and works hard to the best of his abilities to achieve his goals. His interests include reading, sports, film, taking part in outdoor activities and listening to music.

Facebook.com/BayanAzizi